Ready Romance

HOT LIPS,
GREAT ESCAPES
& *89* MORE
WAYS to KEEP
LOVE ALIVE

LESLIE & JIMMY CAPLAN
WITH ILLUSTRATIONS BY MARI GAYATRI STEIN

NEW WORLD LIBRARY
NOVATO, CALIFORNIA

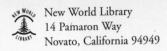

New World Library
14 Pamaron Way
Novato, California 94949

Front cover design by Miller Media
Text design and typography by Mary Ann Casler
Illustrations by Mari Gayatri Stein

Portions of this book were originally published as *Recipes for Romance.*

Library of Congress Cataloging-in-Publication Data
Caplan, Leslie,
Ready for romance : hot lips, great escapes, & 89 other
enticing recipes for keeping love alive / by Leslie and Jimmy Caplan.
p.   cm.
Rev. ed. of: Recipes for romance. © 1996.
ISBN 1-57731-238-4
1. Man-woman relationships. 2. Sexual excitement. 3. Love. 4.
Intimacy (Psychology) I. Caplan, Jimmy, II. Caplan, Leslie,
Recipes for romance. III. Title.

306.7—dc21   2002151072
First Printing, January 2003
ISBN 1-57731-238-4
Printed in Canada on acid-free, partially recycled paper
Distributed to the trade by Publishers Group West
10 9 8 7 6 5 4 3 2 1

To our children
David, Kelly, Gillian, and Kian —

*You have made this journey richer and more romantic
than we ever thought possible.*

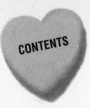

CONTENTS

Zensational

Deep Impressions

Special Deliveries

A Breath of Fresh Air

Beyond the Two of Us

Naughty 'n' Nice

Somewhere in Time

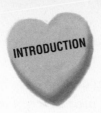
INTRODUCTION

When we first met and fell in love, Leslie was a single parent mom and Jimmy was a bachelor, never before married. As our relationship developed, we began to wonder if our love could continue to grow and develop indefinitely; or, as with our former relationships, it would dissipate over time and eventually lead to our breakup. Rather than overly debate this question, we thought out loud, "What can we do to strengthen our love and enjoy greater romance over time?"

A number of excellent books, tapes, and relationship seminars helped, but the most instructive thing we did was to spend a lot of time interviewing and socializing with close couples — those we knew to be deeply in love after being together for as many as fifty years. Their generous and open responses to our many questions about sustaining romance, along with the inspiration we felt just by being around them, touched us deeply and formed the basis of our previous book, *Recipes for Romance*.

Since the publication of that book, our family has grown to include four children, increasing the demands of parenthood, and challenging our best intentions to keep our romance as strong as it began. We were giving so much time to the children that there was little time left for us to be alone. And when we were able to carve out a date night, we would default to a familiar routine like dinner and a movie. As the kids got a little older, however, we regained some flexibility, and we felt the need to revive our creativity and find novel ways to express our passion. We knew it was time to go back to the drawing board, but this time in a more comprehensive way.

Spurred by our insatiable curiosity — and aided by several wonderful babysitters — we embarked on one of the most satisfying and enriching chapters of our marriage. All the extensive hours of writing this book, pushing each other's creativity, and trying out fresh recipes has been a romantic joyride, bringing us closer together than ever before. And getting to know and share stories with other incurable romantics has been much more fun than work. Today, whether the babysitter stays with our kids at home or takes them out on an adventure so we can be at home alone, we have many wonderful options to consider.

We are thrilled that *Ready for Romance* goes far beyond our earlier observations about keeping love alive. It offers exciting new recipes and includes sample servings from a much larger population of couples and even some romantic singles. There are numerous websites and other references cited throughout to help you plan your own romantic escapades. And each section of the book focuses on specific relationship needs and addresses them in a straightforward and playful manner. Zensational, for example, suggests ways of being romantic that strengthen communications; Breaking Boundaries has some wonderful examples of how to stretch and grow through romance; Naughty 'n' Nice is an adult section that offers tasteful insights for creating those most private moments; and, in The Write Stuff, accomplished creative writers serve up their own special recommendations for love and romance.

The recipes in this book cover a wide range of activities, from simple gestures to elaborate plans. It doesn't matter whether you've just met someone, or have been a couple for many years and are looking for ways to instigate more passion; you'll find a number of enticing things to do at any stage of your relationship. Whether you do these things for one another indoors or outdoors, alone with your mate or in the company of others, you only need to start turning the pages that follow to begin a thoroughly enjoyable and enriching gourmet treat.

So...experiment. Have fun! There's no longer any excuse for you to be unprepared for love. It's time to get *Ready for Romance!*

The Spice of Life

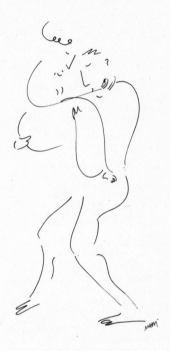

To love and be loved is to feel the sun from both sides.

— David Viscott

1. Hot Lips

Whoever named it necking was a poor judge of anatomy.

— Groucho Marx

I wasn't kissing her. I was whispering in her mouth.

— Chico Marx

❧ Sweet breath
❧ 15 to 20 seconds

*S*urprise your partner with a long hug and kiss (fifteen to twenty seconds) that is not a part of foreplay. Relax into each other's embrace and enjoy the togetherness. No dressing up, planning, or budgeting is required, and the benefits are immediate.

When asked for the secret to their long-lasting marriage, a couple married for seventy years responded, "When we kiss, we kiss for a long time." Follow their example and make Hot Lips a minimum daily requirement for your relationship.

If you and your partner are zealous overachievers and want to go for the gold in kissing, you might be interested to know what the competition did: a Vineland, New Jersey, couple is in the *Guinness Book of World Records* for the world's longest kiss: thirty hours, fifty-nine minutes, and twenty-seven seconds. They did it without separating their lips, sitting, eating or drinking, or taking bathroom breaks. Good luck!

2. Love Essentials

Love is not only a feeling, it is also an art.

— Honoré de Balzac

- 🌱 1 or 2 stockpiles of surprises
- 🌱 1 or 2 romantic idea folders
- 🌱 Willingness to transform your bedroom
- 🌱 1 or more books on *Feng Shui* (recommended)
- 🌱 Ability to keep hi-tech in check

omance is like a great meal; it requires proper ingredients and adequate preparation. There are loving habits you can begin to develop now that will nurture your relationship for many years to come. The following preparations will get you started:

- One: Develop a stockpile of surprises: romantic cards and gifts, stationery, decorative pens, wrapping paper, scented candles, massage oil, and romantic music CDs. Retail stores are filled with romantic items around Valentine's Day.
- Two: Start a romantic idea folder. When you see a notice in the newspaper about a concert, play, or lecture

your partner would enjoy, clip it. Other things to add to your folder might be write-ups on new restaurants, weekend get-aways, or art exhibits. All of these can be utilized at a later time or be the foundation for a fabulous date. For example, Jimmy had adored chimpanzees since he was very young, but he had never gotten to hold one. Leslie came across an article about a nearby ranch that trains chimpanzees and other animals for the movies and allows interactive visits and feedings. She put that in her folder and used it later to create a memorable surprise for Jimmy.

- Three: Take a closer look at your bedroom. Make sure it is a soothing, restful environment that promotes intimacy. Pay attention to the colors and fabrics you have chosen and how they affect your senses. Warmer colors are more welcoming and sexually stimulating. Sensual fabrics include satin, velvet, chenille, flannel, silk, and cotton. Every object in the room should be pleasing to both of you and have a positive association. There should be a pleasant view from the bed. Some items that detract from serenity, relaxation, and intimacy are: TVs, computers, exercise equipment, and desks stacked with unfinished business. If any of these must remain in the bedroom, cover or screen them from view. For additional guidance in arranging your environment to enhance intimacy, check out books on *Feng Shui*, the ancient Chinese art of placement. Once you have created a romantic sanctuary, you will feel more refreshed and rested each morning and you'll be anxious to rendezvous there more often.

• Four: Reduce your dependency on technology. Hi-tech is a double-edged sword. The Internet has brought the world to our desktops, but it reduces our physical contact with other human beings when overused. Bond with your partner at bedtime instead of connecting with strangers in chat rooms until 2:00 A.M. Cell phones and pagers may keep us closer in touch, but answering calls in the middle of romantic walks, meals, or car rides can interrupt feelings of passion and, in excess, be outright rude. If *we* are spending too much time on the telephone, our older daughter, Kelly, admonishes us, "I'm more important than the phone." And when the family gets into the car, it is not unusual to hear her sister, Gillian, cry out emphatically, "No phoney-baloney."

3. Kick the Habit

*Mix up the ingredients in your life
and nibble on something new.*

- ❦ Desire to change
- ❦ An eye for the unusual
- ❦ 1 schedule, shredded

Is your routine as a couple fairly predictable? Do you tend to favor the same restaurants, activities, and friends? If so, it's time to break out of your mold and start replacing the familiar with the unfamiliar. It's a terrific way to reawaken your partner's interest in you and the relationship and add spontaneity to your daily activities.

There are so many habits to choose from...and play with. Change your hair or clothing style or surprise him in the shower. Plan some activities together, like going for an ethnic food you've never tried, spending the night in a double sleeping bag in front of the fire, having a picnic dinner in bed, camping out in your backyard, walking or biking instead of driving, or taking a yoga class together.

Playing hooky is a mischievous way to bust a rut. S̶time with your partner when you normally wouldn't together. Take a day or half-day off from work; skip a class, shopping trip, or weekly card game. Tell him that he's more important than your scheduled plans, and show you mean it by doing something both of you will enjoy. At first you may feel a little guilty being away from the office or your usual companions. However, making her top priority can reawaken feelings of spontaneity and excitement that help keep the relationship fresh. It will also encourage you to keep each other at the top of your daily planning lists.

onic Convergence

At the touch of love everyone becomes a poet.

— Plato

- ❦ 1 secluded setting
- ❦ Writing materials
- ❦ Artful brainstorming
- ❦ Skillful collaboration

*C*reate or find an area inside or outside your home where you and your partner will be undisturbed. Choose a subject that interests you both and select a medium to jointly express your creativity on that subject. You can write alternate lines of poetry, compose the music and lyrics of a song, coauthor a screenplay, or start a travel journal as a reminder of your trips together.

This can be done on a onetime or regular basis. Either way, your collaboration could result in something as simple as a greeting in a birthday card, or a poem commemorating a milestone such as a graduation, anniversary, or retirement. It may even evolve into something more elaborate, such as a published book. This process could uncover latent creativity that would otherwise remain unexpressed by one or both of you. If your budding talents are really in sync, it may also be the beginning of an ongoing creative partnership.

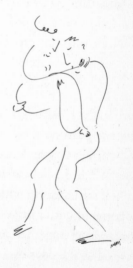

5. Count Me In

Step into your partner's shoes — and walk around a bit.

- ❧ Interest in your partner's interests
- ❧ Availability
- ❧ Desire to tag along

Show how much you care by taking more of an interest in something your partner has usually done without you. Be her caddy on a round of eighteen holes of golf. Assist him when he buys the groceries. Join her at a cooking class. Help him finish the cabinet he's been making in the garage.

Sample Serving

Although I have an aversion to shopping, it is Leslie's favorite pastime. One Saturday morning I got caught up in her enthusiasm and decided to accompany her to a garage sale. While Leslie searched for overlooked treasures, I found myself schmoozing with the sellers, and in the end I actually negotiated better prices on Leslie's purchases. Now we go to garage sales together on a fairly regular basis, and I get as excited as she does over great finds for our house and family.

6. Two Scents' Worth

Spend a little more time with this aromatic aphrodisiac.

- 1 well-stocked perfume counter
- Susceptibility to irresistibility
- Essential oils and accessories (recommended)
- 1 reference book on aromatherapy (recommended)

Go together to a great perfume counter and try on many fragrances until you each find a new perfume or cologne that you both really like. You may want to purchase compatible his and her fragrances by the same designer; they often complement each other well. Wear these scents for special occasions, romantic adventures, or lovemaking. They can serve as olfactory aphrodisiacs, triggering strong emotions associated with these experiences and being a powerful turn-on.

Once you observe the power of fragrance, you may want to become a perfumer for your own body and home. It's really quite easy. Visit an essential oil counter at a pharmacy or health store. Buy the oils that appeal to you and learn about various ways to spread the scents. An easy way to get ited is to make a spray by mixing eighteen drops of your oil into a two-ounce, dark glass spray bottle; fill it with purified water, close, shake, and it's ready for use. Experiment by misting your selected scents around different rooms, on freshly laundered sheets and pillowcases, and on your body. This mixing-and-matching will help maintain a heightened sense of smell. To discover more about the therapeutic benefits and romantic uses of essential oils, refer to one of the many books available on aromatherapy.

7. Partners in Passion

One of life's greatest luxuries is to be passionate about something with someone you are passionate about.

- ❦ 1 shared hobby interest
- ❦ A love of the hunt
- ❦ Long-term commitment

One activity that offers delightful bonding time for couples is exploring a hobby that involves collectibles. It may spring from a common interest that attracted you to each other at the beginning of your relationship, or perhaps it will be something you discover together. Examples are art, antiques, books, wine, figurines or miniatures, plants, vintage photographs and other memorabilia, or stuffed animals.

Once you embark on your chosen path, there are a number of activities that can deepen your knowledge on the subject and add to the pleasure of collecting: subscribing to magazines and newsletters; attending classes, seminars, and auctions; joining clubs; hosting and attending gatherings with other people who share your interests. Some hobbyists like to plan vacations that include tours and dedicated shopping to feed their passion, or use their buying interest as a great way to break up long car trips. The Internet is an excellent source of commentary and research, and offers auction and e-transaction sites. You may even want to set up your own website so other hobbyists worldwide can contact you directly.

If your relationship seems a bit stagnant, consider Partners in Passion as a way of pushing you in a direction that sparks new interest and enthusiasm. A simple inquiry can ripen into a lifetime adventure.

Sample Serving

A friend of ours who owns a nursery told us he regularly assists couples in expanding plant collections that reflect a variety of themes, such as biblical (any plant mentioned in the Bible), tropical, and medicinal. Another couple that likes to travel often has developed a vacation memento collection. In every city and special location they visit, they search for a single perfect reminder that costs no more than five dollars. Over the past ten years, they have accumulated more than fifty meaningful items, including magnets, key chains, aprons, shot glasses, paperweights, pennants, and postcards.

It was unlikely that Shaun and Kareen would ever meet. They lived in different parts of the country and were pursuing different careers. Yet a common bond brought them together. Shaun, the president of a public company, enjoyed gourmet dining and collected fine wines. Kareen was an active attorney, fabulous cook, and wine enthusiast. Shaun put out a profile of himself on America Online and actively sought a mate by looking at other people's profiles. When he saw Kareen's, her passion for food and wine intrigued him, and he sent her an e-mail introducing himself. Kareen did not respond to the communication; so he waited until he saw she was online, and contacted her via *instant messenger*. His inquiry was a single question, "So how much do you like wine?"

That one overture led to several months of e-mail correspondence. Eventually they traded photos and began conversing by phone. The thousand miles that separated them was finally eliminated when they met for dinner at the home of one of her relatives. All went well; Shaun brought three great vintages of French and California wine, and Kareen made a fabulous dinner. They decided to pursue a long-distance relationship and married one year later.

Today Shaun and Kareen love the thrill of searching for great wines. They visit many renowned wineries and take pride in discovering smaller, lesser-known ones. They have developed an extensive wine cellar and enjoy every opportunity to sit quietly and open a great bottle of vintage wine. They discuss the region of the world where the wine came from, its special attributes, and the current affairs of the day when the wine was produced. Kareen also researches the food that complements that particular bottle, and prepares the meal accordingly.

The only thing Shaun and Kareen enjoy more than dining alone is sharing their passion with family and friends. They regularly host intimate gatherings where they serve fine wines and delicious foods. They love acquainting good company with the taste and knowledge of such culinary delights, and gaining added insight from other aficionados who may be present. In every case, a good time is had by all.

$8.$ Poetry in Motion

Dancing is the art of physical poetry. You express yourself with your body rather than words.

— Doyle Barnett

- ❦ 4 feet with a beat
- ❦ Dance lessons (optional)

The music is seductive. You can just sit or stand there, watch, hum, sing along, or let your body become an instrument in the song, so expressive and compelling that it pulls your partner — and perhaps others — along with you. Dancing is one of the easiest and most direct ways to physically communicate and connect with each other. It offers an instant bonding experience, which explains why so many different forms of dance continue to captivate the hearts of young and seasoned lovers alike.

There is something about dancing that helps you become more confident and less self-conscious. Whether you're in the kitchen or bedroom, on the sidewalk or street, at a restaurant or party, moving your bodies together makes a romantic statement, "We are acting as one. We love being together. Whatever other people may think does not concern us." Poetry in Motion frees you from both inhibition and intimidation.

If you're already familiar with this recipe, you know how powerful it can be for promoting intimacy. Freestyle dancing to rock 'n' roll, hip-hop, rave, or jungle music costs nothing and can be done in a bar or club or wherever you are right now. A few introductory lessons can familiarize you with the joy of folk, ethnic (polka, line), and ballroom dancing. There is smooth ballroom (waltz, fox-trot, tango) and Latin, or rhythm (cha-cha, rumba, swing, hustle, mambo, merengue). But be advised up front: many couples who sign up for a few lessons to learn some steps so they won't look foolish at an upcoming dance or reception end up taking regular classes for many months or even years.

Whether you are alone in the rain (recipe 44: Wet Dreams) or one of hundreds of couples at a New Year's Eve ball (recipe 88: The Possible Dream), dancing can be meditative, inspirational, sensual, or sexual, but it is never boring. It's also great and invigorating exercise. Treat yourself to a few minutes — or a lifetime — of this exhilarating activity. You may also meet some wonderful new friends along the way.

9. Spa Day

The saddest thing I can imagine is to get used to luxury.

— Charlie Chaplin

- ❦ Freedom from all responsibilities
- ❦ Permission to be partners-in-hedonism
- ❦ Appointment with yourselves (1-day minimum)
- ❦ 1 upscale spa with pool, sauna, and Jacuzzi (preferred)
- ❦ 2 to 3 treatments
- ❦ Babysitter for kids or pets (if applicable)
- ❦ 1 hotel/spa package (highly recommended)

Sometimes you just have to get away from it all and splurge a little on yourselves. And if you and your lover want a day to remember that is easy to plan, you're in luck. It's closer than you think, and the benefits are immediate: physical and mental rejuvenation, increased circulation and flexibility, stress-free relaxation, and time to be intimate.

Make a local day spa or hotel spa your home for the entire day. Choose one in your area that is known for offering many different types of treatments in a luxurious setting.

Call ahead and ask if the spa will allow you, at no additional cost, to relax all day and use its facilities (pool, sauna, steam room, Jacuzzi, guest lounge) when you book treatments there. Most spas have facial and body treatments as well as various types of massage therapy. Decide on those that sound the most appealing and schedule two or more for each of you during your Spa Day.

Arrive early and bring only a bathing suit. Take off all your clothes and put on bathrobes provided by the spa. If you don't know it already, hanging out in a bathrobe all day can be a liberating experience. In between your scheduled treatments, you may want to read, meditate, or have a light meal when not using the spa's facilities. At the end of a day like this, the only question will be, "How soon can we come back?"

If you want to push the envelope of relaxation even further, consider booking a one- or two-night hotel/spa combination package. These are offered by many hotel spas, and prices are usually quite reasonable when packages are booked during the slower days, Monday through Thursday. This means the spa will be less crowded, which translates into a more tranquil environment. And you also have the option of periodically going back to your own room in addition to resting by the pool, taking a Jacuzzi, and sweating out toxins in the sauna or steam bath. Be sure to have enough time between treatments throughout the day so you can enjoy all these benefits without feeling rushed.

The best thing about booking the combination package

is that you don't have to leave the spa in the late afternoon or evening and get into your car and deal with traffic. That can be quite a contrast. Wouldn't it be sweeter to finish your last massages, walk hand-in-hand back to your luxurious room, and spend the rest of the evening undisturbed — except, perhaps, for the brief interruption of room service? Imagine the high level of passion and eroticism that can be created by two completely relaxed and rejuvenated loving bodies.

Sample Serving

Lou and Gloria had spent months planning and preparing for their formal wedding. In the midst of the stress and jitters, Lou informed Gloria that she should not make any plans on the Thursday before their wedding weekend. That would be designated as "their day."

That Thursday finally arrived and Lou took Gloria to a local hotel, where they treated themselves to a poolside breakfast. It was a warm, sunny morning and they enjoyed fresh fruit, juices, and an array of tasty muffins under an umbrella. They talked and read without any distractions until noon, when Lou escorted Gloria to the hotel's spa facility. He had arranged a full day of joint relaxation and pampering, beginning with a manicure, pedicure, and hand massage. They alternated treatments with visits to the sauna and Jacuzzi, where toxins and impurities just melted from their bodies. After a cool, refreshing shower, they donned fluffy robes and rested in the spa's spacious lounge, where they rehydrated themselves with herbal ice teas and imported bottled water.

Now Lou and Gloria were ready for the last leg of their pleasure journey. Two masseuses arrived to escort them to a private room for a couple's massage, where they breathed the aromatic fragrances Lou had chosen and were soothed by the many candles and soft music. Together they drifted in and out of consciousness while enjoying their full-body massages. For Lou, the ultimate pleasure was being able to look over and lock eyes with the most important person in his universe and feel their souls unite.

As their Spa Day came to an end, Lou and Gloria felt revitalized, renewed in energy and spirit, and ready to face the biggest day of their lives.

10. The Great Escape

Regular gourmet treats are a necessity of life.

❦ Any excuse to get away
❦ The good sense to leave the world behind

*T*ake a mini-vacation at least once every two months — just get away. Waiting for the one or two weeks next year can snowball into a mountain of anxiety. You don't have to fly away to Rio or the Bahamas to relax. Take advantage of a weekend special at a local hotel or bed-and-breakfast inn; don't be afraid to request the honeymoon package. You can also take a train trip, rent a houseboat or yacht, or go camping in a romantic setting (see recipe 69: Roughing It).

Sample Serving

Diane loves art. Her father was a portrait painter and her husband, Ralph, is a successful landscape artist who also owns and operates an art gallery in Santa Barbara. Several times each year, they take weekend trips to different spots along the California coast such as Carmel and Laguna Beach. They favor those places which boast romantic lodging, a leisurely pace, excellent restaurants, and, most important, good art.

One of their favorite getaways is a delightful working vacation that occurs every summer at the California Art Club Competition in Mission San Juan Capistrano. Ralph and many other talented artists will arrive on a Monday in mid-August and begin painting the gorgeous grounds of the Mission from dawn to dusk over the next several days. They are inspired by the Mission's old-world character and charm, and their creative output will be displayed and sold at a much anticipated art show on Saturday and Sunday.

Diane takes the train and joins Ralph at midweek so they do not have to return home in separate vehicles. They stay at a hotel directly across from the Mission, so it's easy for Ralph to take his art supplies back and forth. As Ralph paints, Diane enjoys a visual feast as she walks among the artists at work. She marvels at their respective approaches and is continually reminded that in every nook and cranny lurks a beautiful painting.

Ralph and Diane welcome this yearly event as a kind of spiritual renewal. They can relax without distractions and enjoy the camaraderie of other artists, many of whom return every year. They discuss the art market, other painters they admire, future shows not to miss, and galleries to visit. If, at the weekend art show, Ralph has sold some of his plein air paintings to admiring attendees, he will be able to cover part to all of his costs for the entire week. Both Ralph and Diane feel that receiving any money for that much enjoyment is just icing on the cake.

Mark Twain once commented that success is when your vocation becomes your vacation. Ralph and Diane have created a life that certainly lives up to this ideal.

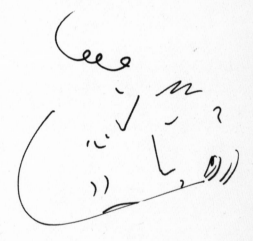

Some Enchanted Evening

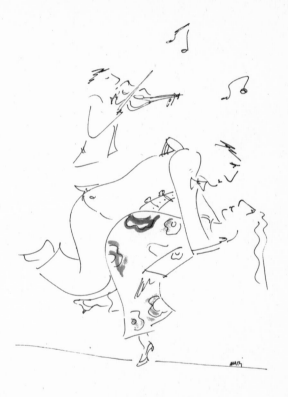

Too much of a good thing can be wonderful.

— Mae West

11. Date Night

*One of the best and most often ignored ways of
keeping your relationship novel and exciting.*

- ❦ 1 night alone with each other every week
- ❦ 2 large helpings of creativity
- ❦ Receptivity to change
- ❦ Willingness to take turns

*D*on't let yourself be boxed into the "dinner-movie-home to bed" routine. Get out and exercise your creativity. Choose one night each week that belongs to the two of you and take turns planning the date. Try some of the ideas suggested in this book or dream up some of your own.

This recipe produces the best results when you are receptive to each other's requests, even if your mate asks you to go along with something you would normally not be inclined to do. Think of it as an opportunity to try something new and gain additional insight into your respective tastes and preferences.

Practice Date Night regularly and you will have some nice surprises along the way. Two of our friends have faithfully kept up this practice over the course of their twenty-year marriage, and the husband tells us he often enjoys the evenings his wife plans more than his own. Another couple we know has had what they call an "affair" almost every Wednesday afternoon during their fifty years of marriage. Memories of their romantic escapades, which range from afternoon tea dancing to trysts at adult motels, are better than some people's fantasies and demonstrate the cumulative value of Date Night.

12. Surprise Date

A great way to whet your partner's appetite!

- 2 show tickets (or invitation to dinner)
- 1 familiar place
- 1 envelope and pen
- 1 to 2 decorative magnets (optional)
- 1 blindfold (alternative)
- Ability to keep a secret

*P*lace show tickets or an invitation to dinner or special event inside an envelope. Write a brief message on the outside of the envelope, for example: "Surprise for my Hottie" or "Big things come in small packages."

Be sure to put the envelope in an area where it will be readily noticed. Leave it by the computer, tape it to the bathroom mirror, or secure it on the refrigerator with a decorative magnet or embossed photo.

An alternative is to blindfold your partner and take him to an undisclosed location. He will quickly lose his sense of direction and probably ask a lot of questions as he wonders what you possibly could have planned. Do your best to be sure the surprise at the end of the ride meets or exceeds the anticipation.

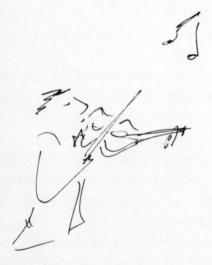

13. Progressive Dining

Food for thought... and action!

❦ 2 big appetites
❦ 3 to 4 restaurants

$\mathcal{T}$his recipe provides great food, the perfect ambience, and there's no cleanup!

Most people enjoy dining out; it often plays a big part in the romantic experience. Some of our best memories may involve food, particularly those occasions when we ventured out and tried something different. Such an important part of life and romance should never lose its sense of adventure and become routine. One of our favorite ways to revive variety, playfulness, and intimacy is to stage a progressive dinner. It's as easy as going to an area of your town — or a place you are visiting — where there is a concentration of excellent restaurants. Walk around with your partner, check out some menus, and discuss which ones interest you most. It's okay to consider ones with which you are already familiar, but favor some new options as well.

Now go into one of your preferred choices and explain to the host or hostess that you are doing a progressive dinner among several restaurants that evening. Relax with a drink and order an appetizer. Afterward, move on to the second restaurant or bistro for soup or salad, then to a third for the main course, and follow up with a fourth for dessert; or change the order to accommodate your preferences. Be sure to walk around between courses and admire the scenery or do some window-shopping. You may want to enjoy coffee, tea, or an evening drink at an inviting café before heading home or going off to some late-night engagement.

Progressive Dining enables you to broaden the menu and savor a variety of tastes. It's also a healthier way to eat because you pace your intake of food and drink and promote better digestion when walking between locations. At first, you may feel a little awkward about explaining your intentions to the host or hostess, but don't let that hold you back. Most will respond with warmth and enthusiasm.

Sample Serving

Leslie once used the progressive dinner theme to create one of the most memorable evenings of my life. On the day before one of my birthdays, she encouraged me to go for a leisurely workout, sauna, and shower before coming home to a special meal she was preparing. When I came back to the house, however, there was a note on the back door. I will never forget Leslie's instructions: "The kids are handled. Take off all your clothes and meet me in the bedroom."

It was like a scene out of a comedy movie. I was so excited that I started undressing as I dashed through the house, only to trip halfway up the stairs and take a terrible fall. Aching but undeterred, I got to the top of the landing, took off what was left of my clothing and burst through the bedroom door. Imagine my surprise when I found the room empty. I would have felt like the victim of a practical joke, were it not for gifts she had left me.

Laid out on the bed was a new outfit from my favorite store, socks and underwear included. Propped inside a coiled new belt was a card that told me to get dressed immediately and walk down our street exactly three blocks to find Leslie. I did as I was instructed, and found my sweetie inside a romantic booth at a European restaurant, which was part of a Victorian bed-and-breakfast. She had arranged for the chef to start making my favorite appetizer — shrimp-and-scallop cakes — when I walked through the door.

It was a warm summer evening, and we were excited about our quest for progressive culinary satisfaction. We next enjoyed salad from the outdoor second-floor balcony of a Mediterranean bistro, and then proceeded to a popular and very busy Italian restaurant for Chilean sea bass baked in a wood oven. Afterward, we were at first too full to think of dessert, so we took a break by visiting two antique malls and chatting with some shop owners before concluding the evening on the right bite: a swan sculptured from puffed pastry, topped with ice cream and floating on a sea of melted chocolate.

When I look back on that consummate evening, I am touched as much by Leslie's creative setup as by the thrill of enjoying a new approach to dining. It was the best and most delicious birthday eve of my life.

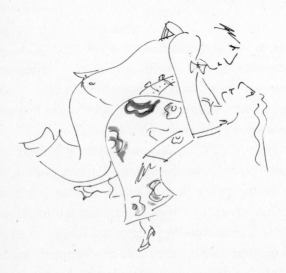

14. Hot Wheels

Adventure is the champagne of life.

— G. K. Chesterton

- ❦ 1 uncommon means of transportation
- ❦ Flowers, special gift, or treat (optional)
- ❦ Shift in perspective

*S*howing up in a rented limousine can be a marvelous surprise in itself or as part of an evening's event, particularly if your loved one has never been treated to that kind of luxury before.

But there are lower-cost, open-air alternatives that have their own unique charm and will add variety and a sense of adventure to any special outing. You're bound to create quite an impression when you arrive to pick up your mate in one of the following: tandem bicycle, bicycle rickshaw or surrey, moped, horse-drawn cart, roller blades, electric mini-car, or golf cart (where not prohibited by law).

Whatever type of wheels you choose, you may want to further enrich the experience by greeting your partner with flowers, a meaningful gift, or romantic treat. One of the delightful results of using uncommon transportation on a date is the opportunity to appreciate your town or the countryside from a different perspective.

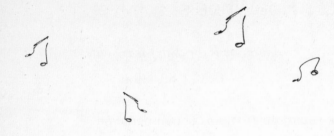

15. Unexpected Anniversary

It all depends on the secret ingredient.

❧ Flexibility to mix up the natural order
❧ 1 generous portion of imagination
❧ 1 or more gifts (optional)
❧ A little help from family and friends (optional)

One of the drawbacks of birthdays, anniversaries, and holidays is that they are set dates; your loved one already expects something to happen at those times. For a nice change, catch him off guard by celebrating the occasion on a date other than the actual one. Or create a surprise anniversary event to commemorate such things as a half-birthday (recipe 73: Talk of the Town), the date he came to town or landed the perfect job, or when you first moved in together.

Staging an Unexpected Anniversary and finding an unusual way to celebrate it will add a shot of vitality to any relationship. It can be a private affair, or include family and friends. Remember, the odder the timing, the greater the impact.

Richard and Eileen like to talk about the traveling they'll do when all four of their children are grown. They can just picture their best friends joining them for ski trips and cruises. So, for their twentieth wedding anniversary, Richard decided to give his lovely bride a taste of their future.

Eileen was thrilled when she heard they were going to Stowe, Vermont, for a mini-vacation at the Topnotch Resort and Spa. The plan was to check in on a Wednesday, the actual day of their anniversary, and then stay through the weekend.

Alone in the car, enjoying the five-hour ride from their home in Connecticut to one of their favorite destinations, Richard and Eileen felt like a young couple again. They arrived on schedule and settled in for a quiet and relaxing weekend. Eileen was flattered by the extra-special attention they received from people at the hotel and at Mr. Pickwick's Pub & Restaurant in Ye Olde England Inne, the scene of their romantic anniversary dinner. Richard promised to take her shopping over the next several days to find the perfect antique to commemorate their twentieth year together.

When they came downstairs for dinner on Friday evening, Richard suggested they check out some of the resort's wonderful little meeting areas and led her to a small, cozy room with a fireplace. When she looked inside, Eileen had quite a shock. Four of their favorite couples were waiting for her by the fireplace. After many hugs and congratulations, Eileen learned that the entire group had come to Top Notch, at Richard's invitation, to help celebrate their anniversary. They had a lot of fun keeping this secret for months and coordinating schedules with Richard earlier that day so they could check in and keep out of sight until dinnertime. Following cocktails and hors d'oeuvres, the group was escorted to a private dining room where the banquet table had been covered with carnations, Eileen's favorite flowers, and twenty long tapered candles. Over wine and good food, ten best friends were able to relax and enjoy the remarkable evening Richard had envisioned.

After thanking everyone for coming to Stowe, Richard turned to Eileen and said, "Many people advised me on what to give you for our twentieth anniversary. Most suggested an expensive necklace, earrings, a tennis bracelet, or watch. However, instead of a piece of jewelry to hang around your neck or wrist, I decided on something special you can wrap around your heart."

16. Strangers in the Night

Love is what makes a crowd disappear
when you're with someone.
— Elvis Presley

- ❧ 1 place with unfamiliar faces
- ❧ Provocative attire
- ❧ Desire to role-play
- ❧ No expectations

*H*ave you ever thought about picking up your partner? That's right, meeting him or her again for the first time.

This works best when you dress up independently of each other and create a "surprise look." If you're living in the same house, perhaps one of you can prepare for the evening elsewhere. For your rendezvous, choose a place where singles meet and where it is unlikely you will run into any of your friends. It could be a bar, dance, or social event. Come separately but at approximately the same time, circulate, and see what happens.

Picking up your partner once or twice a year is a good way to revive the joy of dating and show renewed interest in your partner. No two nights will be the same if you leave your expectations at home.

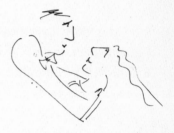

...e Envelope, Please

Your date with fate.

- ❦ 3 cards with envelopes
- ❦ Assortment of decorative pens
- ❦ Your best penmanship
- ❦ Imagination, with style

Do you have trouble making decisions — maybe yes, maybe no?

Put a new twist on decision-making in your relationship, adding laughter and removing angst. Imagine three different types of dates you know your partner would enjoy and write down a colorful description of each one on a separate card. Then, when he asks, "What do you want to do tonight?" surprise him with the envelopes, numbered one, two, and three. "Tonight your fate is sealed. Pick one!"

Don't give him any hints, but you may want to make teasing facial gestures as he examines each envelope. The more he struggles in choosing his destiny, the more fun you will have with this kind of date foreplay. After he makes the big decision, you can go one of two ways: 1. let him open it, and then proceed according to plan; or 2. *you* may insist, first, that you open the other two envelopes and reveal what was hidden inside them before he finds out where his chosen envelope will lead you that night.

Another scenario is to plan something very special and make the contents of all three envelopes the same. After he chooses, put the other two away or destroy them. "The night may have a thousand eyes, but it will never see these!" That should add to the mystery, and start the fun!

18. Unforgettable

*Few of us can do great things, but all of us can
do small things with great love.*

— Mother Teresa

❧ Ability to love unconditionally
❧ Desire to give unconditionally

*T*here is no greater high in life than knowing you have made someone else's life happier or sweeter. True love is more than a feeling. It is making a commitment to the welfare of your partner and letting her know it through words and deeds.

Periodically, arrange a date that shows, by your thoughtful planning, the depth of your feelings. It can serve to raise your partner's spirits when fate has not been kind, highlight a positive development like a promotion or the completion of a project, or celebrate the length of your relationship. Do this recipe with a pure heart. Focus on your intentions; be unattached to the results. Simply enjoy!

Susan and Mark had been happily married for seven years and wanted to have a second child. However, their schedules were so hectic they weren't even taking the time to be romantic. Susan decided to create an unforgettable evening for Mark.

The couple chose a night when their son could have a sleepover with his grandparents and they were free from all other commitments. No specific plans were made; but on the day of the date, Susan called Mark at work and asked him to meet her for drinks at 5:00 P.M. in the bar of an elegant hotel. As she expected, Mark was hesitant. "I don't think so. I don't want to be hanging out in the bar if you're late." Susan promised him she would be on time and, reluctantly, he agreed.

Mark arrived on time, but Susan wasn't there. Annoyed, he resigned himself to a first solo drink, figuring she would get there eventually, and then they could go out for dinner and take in a movie. What he didn't know was that his beautiful wife was ready for romance and anxiously waiting for him in a room upstairs. The problem was that the bartender had forgotten to give Mark an envelope from Susan after he ordered that first drink.

Half an hour passed, and Susan couldn't stand the suspense any longer. She called down to the bar, and an apologetic bartender handed Mark a note that read, "No, I'm not late, and if you use this key you'll be able to find me." Surprised and elated, he hurried to the room.

Whatever Mark may have expected that night, he was blown away when Susan opened the door. There stood his voluptuous bride wearing custom-made sheer lingerie. The music of Joan Armatrading played softly in the background. Susan gave him a passionate kiss and pulled him into the candlelit room, stocked with champagne, caviar, shrimp on ice, and chocolate-dipped strawberries.

The evening did much more than reignite their passion: it made them proud parents again exactly nine months later.

Zensational

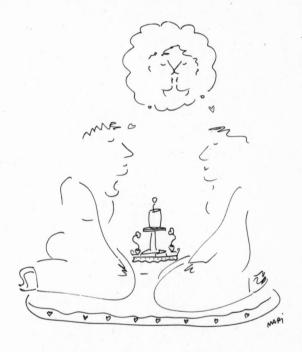

Your presence is required; your presents are not.

19. Heart-to-Heart

Indulge in the sweet sound of your partner's voice.

- ❦ 2 tender voices
- ❦ Food for positive thoughts
- ❦ A little time in a quiet space

*F*alling in love is the term we use to describe the sudden deep connection we experience with another human being. It can be so intoxicating that, in the beginning, the possibility of ever falling out of love is unimaginable. Successful couples know that romance can grow only when those initial feelings of connectedness are recognized and nurtured through communication and caring.

Whenever possible, take about fifteen to twenty minutes before retiring at night to simply be with your partner without any outside distractions. (If this seems daunting, promise yourself that you'll try it for a month, on one designated night a week.) Turn off computers, stereos, and TVs; turn your full attention to each other. It's a great way to stay current by airing differences or concerns, discussing positive ideas and insights, or reviewing interesting stories from books, magazines, or newspaper articles. You may want to recite poetry or serenade your partner. If you are not married or living together, hook up by phone. This is one of those times when instant messaging and e-mail are poor substitutes for the real thing.

Heart-to-Heart is a way of checking in at the end of a long day. It safeguards romance by encouraging you to continue the communication and caring that started at the beginning of your relationship.

20. Easy Listening

I like not only to be loved, but to be told I am loved.

— George Eliot

- ❦ 3 sincere compliments
- ❦ Give and take
- ❦ 1 bed, 2 pillows (optional)

*O*ver time, couples may forget about one of romance's basic rules: express regular praise in a loving manner and keep criticism to a minimum. Not just thinking about but telling your partner the things you admire in him will convey the all-important message, "I don't take this relationship for granted."

Find a few minutes of quiet during the day, or at night before falling asleep, to sit or lie quietly together and comment on three things about him that please you. While it's easy to compliment physical appearance, give it some thought and show additional consideration by focusing on his behavior and character traits. Let her know you've noticed the special things she has said or done. Perhaps he will want to reciprocate immediately afterward, or the next time.

Be sure to state your compliments in a positive light, and accept them graciously when you're on the receiving end. This means acknowledging the praise with a simple "Thank you," nod of appreciation, or gentle kiss. Never downplay what you are being praised for with a comment like, "Ah, it was really nothing."

Not only will your partner find the listening easy and bask in the warmth of your appreciation, but your comments will also remind you of your own good fortune. If done as part of Heart-to-Heart (previous recipe) before going to sleep, it can be the perfect way to end the day!

21. Lighten Up

Humor is emotional chaos remembered in tranquility.

— James Thurber

A cheerful heart is good medicine, but a crushed spirit dries up the bones.

— Proverbs 17:22

❧ 2 spirited dispositions
❧ Ability to laugh, whatever the situation

*I*t's not a laughing matter... and yet it is!

We all go through times when life runs counter to our expectations; even the most romantic couples can have their rough spots. Yet love can be strengthened by every experience, provided we keep our sense of humor and never take ourselves too seriously.

Humor gives us a sense of perspective on our problems, and the therapeutic value of laughter for mental and physical well-being has been medically documented. Whenever we are able to laugh in and *at* the face of adversity, there is an actual shift in our consciousness and an emotional release from the thing that has been troubling us. "If you can laugh at it, you can survive it," advises comedian Bill Cosby.

Be sure your relationship is rich in humor and laughter. They go hand-in-hand with your ability to play and have fun. They serve as stress-busters, allowing you to better appreciate and deal with the incongruities and complexities of modern life. If you are feeling pressured or heavy-hearted and want to work on a way to Lighten Up, consider the following options:

- ❧ Try recipe 45: Play Date
- ❧ Watch a lot of comedy
- ❧ Attend a laughter workshop in your area
- ❧ Visit the Humor Therapy link at holistic-online.com
- ❧ Order tapes of lectures by C.W. Metcalf (our personal favorite)

We asked a long-term Zen practitioner for his insight on humor. "I'm in favor of it," he replied. And his thoughts on laughter? "If something else works, I'm not aware of it."

Sample Servings

Tom and Tina of Spokane, Washington, have been happily married for over twenty years. When Tina heard we were writing this book, she told us that romance for them was not about grand gestures, but rather the everyday things they do for each other. She then put together a list of examples, two of which highlighted the value of humor in a healthy relationship:

• Several years ago, Tom bought Tina a new car and came straight home from the dealer to pick her up so they could go to a formal function. It was a night to remember: they were enjoying the smooth ride and the luxury and smell of the brand-new interior, when suddenly Tina was overwhelmed by a severe case of food poisoning. Before she could even ask Tom to pull over to the side of the road, she vomited all over the car and on her elegant silk dress.

Tom showed his true colors under this most unpleasant circumstance. "Gee, Honey," he said, without missing a beat, "if you didn't like the car, you could have just told me."

• Tina has always loved cooking and preparing special meals for the people she cares about. She and Tom had been dating for several weeks when she decided to show off her talents by inviting him to a delectable meal of shrimp jambalaya, crusty French bread oozing with garlic butter, and a salad of arugula and beefsteak tomatoes with her special chunky blue cheese dressing. For dessert she made blackberry pie, which was to be topped with homemade vanilla ice cream.

Tom was thrilled with the dinner and could hardly wait for dessert. But as Tina was bringing the pie to the table, she tripped on a throw rug. The pie flew out of her hands and landed upside down on the carpet. Without losing her composure, Tina scooped it up, put it back into the pan, and announced, "Well, now we are having blackberry cobbler!"

Tom told her later that anyone who could handle that type of calamity so calmly and turn the situation into something humorous was someone he definitely wanted in his life. And that, she tells us, is the real reason Tom decided to marry her.

Those who laugh, last!

22. The Last Goodbye

Never let the sun set on your anger.

❦ Willingness to take an extra minute
❦ Expressions from the heart

If tragedy struck, and you and your partner could never be together again, how would the survivor reflect on that very last encounter? With fondness, or with uneasy feelings of guilt and regret?

Life is unpredictable. The reality is that whenever we say "goodbye" or "goodnight" to a friend or loved one, there may not be a next time. Therefore, every time you part company, prepare to hang up the phone, or send off an e-mail, be sure to end on a good note. This may include the use of a pet phrase or nickname, a special touch, or simply gazing into each other's eyes.

"Never carry a fight overnight" is a mantra for good health and proper love maintenance. No matter how rushed you or your partner may feel at the moment of departure, it only takes a minute or less to make sure that the last impression is a loving one. If there are any unresolved conflicts, assure your partner you will give her a generous ear and work things out as soon as you get together again. Following this simple ritual communicates a powerful message, "I love you and I'm always with you."

As you become more attentive to The Last Goodbye, start paying attention to the way you say "good morning" or "hello" to your partner as well. Even if he is forty-five minutes late, or returns home without doing the errand he promised not to forget, always greet your partner with warmth and appreciation. Express any necessary grievances a little later in a caring way...before you whack him over the head!

Sample Serving

During their fifty years of marriage, Mike and Jennie have honored their vow to never let the sun *rise* on their anger. No matter how grouchy or upset one or both of them may feel when they get into bed, sometime during the night they *must* touch toes.

23. Do Not Disturb

Sleep dwell upon thine eyes, peace in thy breast.
— William Shakespeare, *Romeo and Juliet*

- 1 sleeping partner
- 1 attentive partner
- Ability to let time unwind

*A*h, the joy of a good night's sleep, or even the opportunity to get a much-needed rest during the day. If your mate is overtired or exhausted and really needs to sleep in or take a long nap, make sure she gets it — all of it. Stay by her, in the bedroom or car, by the pool or the ocean. You can read or write, do some handwork, or just sit quietly and meditate. Part of the time you may want to just look at her and reflect on the relationship, your history together, and common goals for the future.

When she finally decides it's time to get up, be responsive to her needs. Your help in creating a gentle transition from a restful sleep to the world of action will be greatly appreciated. Remember, lovers are unlikely to feel romantic when they're tired or grouchy.

Sample Serving

About six months after they met, Skip and Debbie decided to go to an outdoor film festival to see *Grease*. They chose an excellent spot, laid out their blanket, and got comfortable as they waited for the movie to start. By the time it began, there were more than a thousand people in attendance.

Debbie said she had been quite tired that day, and even her intense interest in the film could not prevent her from falling asleep about an hour after it started. When she awakened at midnight, the crowd had long disappeared. Skip had patiently waited for her to get up on her own rather than disturb her peaceful sleep. He just smiled and asked her if she was ready to go home.

Debbie wondered how many men (or women) would have watched all the other people leave and just waited until their partner awakened. "Not many," she thought, "but I have someone very special who did that for me." Debbie says that, over the years, Skip has never lost the knack of surprising her with endearing romantic gestures.

24. Sabbath Day

If the Lord could find the time, so can you!

- 1 day of quiet time
- Freedom from distractions
- Trusting simplicity
- Asking the right questions
- Meditation time (optional)

Everyone needs time to pause and reflect. Going inward on a regular basis helps revitalize mind, body, and spirit. Similarly, your love life can benefit immensely if you periodically dedicate an entire day to recharging your relationship batteries and clarifying communications with your partner.

Take care of all necessary errands before the chosen day so you will not be distracted. Think about substituting phones, TVs, and computers with nature and/or silence. The mantra of the day is *simplicity:* read, meditate, talk, walk instead of ride, eat simply. Let the moment, not an agenda, guide you. This can also be a beautiful time of reflection: What are our inner needs? Are we on the right path in life? What longings within ourselves have we not addressed? Are we living in harmony with our highest good?

Even if you have your own meditation practice, you may want to experiment with a couple's form of meditation that we affectionately call Zen Sex. Start by sitting comfortably, opposite each other, and gaze into each other's eyes, holding hands if you like. Innocence is the key. Don't try to communicate anything specific, create a special mood, or feel a certain way. Let come what may: thoughts, emotions, tears, laughter. If you don't feel anything at all, that's okay, too. The significance here is that even if you do this exercise only once, you have established an intimate level of just being together; and it will be with you, in a real yet subtle way, at the core of all your other experiences.

Sabbath Day provides a spiritual rest that *should* be taken lightly. In the relaxation and quietness of your extended time together, your busy lives will slow down and regain harmony and balance.

25. The Pleasure List

Do unto others as they want to be done unto.

- ❦ 2 sheets of paper
- ❦ 2 pens
- ❦ Clarity of desire
- ❦ 4 ears wide open

The Golden Rule is beautiful in spirit, but if you treat your loved one the way *you* want to be treated, don't always expect a big thank you. This principle is illustrated by the time Jimmy gave Leslie a rice cooker for their first anniversary. He couldn't understand why she broke down and cried until she explained that while the gift was functional, she feared it might also be symbolic of the end of their romance.

When you follow the Platinum Rule, "Do unto others as they want to be done unto," you satisfy your partner in many different ways because you are aware of and capable of giving her what turns her on, not what you think should turn her on or *what turns you on*. The rice cooker incident brought this principle to light for us, and we began to work on improving our communications. In the process, we developed a remarkably simple exercise that has since helped us avoid unmindful blunders in planning dates, surprises, and in selecting gifts. It's called The Pleasure List.

We each took a piece of paper and listed ten things that always gave us pleasure. Then we exchanged lists and reviewed them out loud to make sure we fully understood each other's needs. That's it! The fifteen minutes it took to do this provided remarkable insight into our individual preferences and stimulated fresh ideas for new romantic adventures. We highly recommend The Pleasure List and suggest you use it periodically, as shifting dynamics in your personal life or relationship may cause your priorities to change over time.

Always be mindful of the Platinum Rule. It's more than a recommendation for life, love, and romance; it's a requirement. You may want to combine it with the next recipe, Honor Thy Lover, to keep your relationship on the fast track of growth.

Sample Serving

Pleasures are not always compatible: Jimmy loves being home all day and co-parenting our young children; he would also like to have more time away from the family to play sports. It can be a source of conflict for him, and I like it when I can do something about it.

Jimmy had been longing for an afternoon of golf with his friend, Steve, so I decided to facilitate a play date he would always remember. One evening I casually mentioned

I had a romantic surprise for him the next afternoon. The babysitting was arranged and everything else had been handled. He was overly curious about what I had planned. Each question was answered only with a smile. As departure time approached, I laid out the ground rules: Jimmy would be blindfolded and led to the car in silence. He was to remain silent until the blindfold was removed.

Just before zero hour, I quickly sprayed my perfume in the car and inserted one of his favorite CDs. A few other items were placed in the trunk. Jimmy was excited as I wrapped a scarf around his eyes and led him to the garage. Once I had helped him into the car and fastened the seat belt, I winked at his friend, Steve, standing nearby. He quietly entered and started the car, and turned on the music. With two sets of golf clubs in the trunk, they headed off to a golf course where I had prepaid a round of eighteen holes for the two of them. (Steve later told me he was a little worried that Jimmy might reach over and try to hold his hand during the twenty-minute ride. Lucky for Steve, Jimmy took advantage of the time to meditate.) He was amazed when the blindfold was removed, and he saw Steve in front of him and the golf course behind him. A bit confused, he looked around for me, and then learned the details of the afternoon plan from Steve.

That evening, Jimmy told me he thought of the entire day as a wonderful, refreshing gift that came at a time when he needed it most.

26. Honor Thy Lover

*Seek to improve yourself and seek the best
interests of the other, not the other way around.*

— Josh McDowell, *The Secret of Loving*

*When a man spends his time giving his wife criticism
and advice instead of compliments, he forgets that
it was not his good judgment, but his charming
manners, that won her heart.*

— Connie Rowland, *Reflections of a Bachelor Girl*

❧ Commitment to growth
❧ Willingness to change for your partner

You fall in love. You adore everything about your partner. The world is perfect. Then, a little farther up the road, when your individual differences start to become more visible and may even clash, you recognize that this match made in Heaven will require some serious attention here on Earth. You may have your arguments and your ups and downs —

that's natural. But love can survive adversity as long as you and your mate know that, at the end of the day, *you are there for each other* — without any qualifications.

Don't fall into the trap of thinking your relationship would be better and you would be happier if only your partner would change this or that. First, it will never make you happy; you'll only keep on finding additional things you want to have fixed. Second, it's not going to happen anyway.

What *should* you do? Turn the tables. In the spirit of "it's better to give than to receive," offer your partner the ultimate gift: ask what it is *you* could do better or change about yourself that would make your loved one happier. The response may surprise you and initiate an honest dialogue that takes the relationship to a new level of intimacy.

Because Honor Thy Lover is a sincere approach to resolving conflict, your gesture will often be reciprocated. And that will initiate a pattern for dealing with disagreements in the future in which both parties take responsibility. Instead of complaining, blaming, or trying to eliminate differences, just ask, "What must we do together to create a solution that harmonizes our differences?"

Sample Serving

Anthony already knew the response he would get to this question. "Be on time; I hate it when we're always late," said Justine. The interesting thing about this dynamic was that, during the many years of their marriage, Anthony felt he had caused them to be late only a few times. Somehow, though, Justine felt tremendous pressure when she wanted to get out the door — particularly as the babysitter arrived — and Anthony was dawdling or doing something that had no immediate importance. Instead of arguing the issue, Anthony was sympathetic and committed to making sure he was ready when Justine was anxious to leave.

A couple weeks later, not yet completely satisfied but secretly thrilled that Anthony was making an effort to cooperate, Justine asked him what it was she could do to make him happier. His answer caught her off guard. The thing he desired most was to be greeted with hugs and kisses whenever he walked through the door. Anthony wanted from Justine the same treatment he got regularly from the children. "I know that sometimes you're overwhelmed and stressed, or upset with me about something," he told her. "But, please, don't dump on me when I first walk in the door. First, show me how much I am loved and appreciated; then it will be easier for me to help you get a handle on things a few minutes later."

Anthony and Justine learned something invaluable about relationships from this experience: Whenever you get into an argument and negative emotions start to escalate, step back and ask yourselves, "What's the real issue here? Why am I really upset?" Many times, what we think we're fighting about and the actual cause of the fight can be very different. It's a case of mistaking the smoke for the fire.

27. Just Hangin'

Is not this the true romantic feeling — not the desire to escape life, but to prevent life from escaping you?

— Thomas Clayton Wolfe

❦ Nothing; absolutely, positively nothing
❦ Ability to take it as it comes

Remember *Seinfeld*, the TV show that prided itself on being about nothing? When was the last time you and your loved one allowed yourselves the luxury of pure indulgence, doing nothing other than what interested you at the moment, unclouded by shoulds and should nots? What makes Just Hangin' different from all the other recipes in Zensational is that it does not have a communications or service agenda. Nor does it require any preparation or exclusions. It is meant to encourage you and your mate to give full attention to whatever is at hand, without feelings of guilt or the fear of being late or missing out on something else. Pretend that the clock does not exist during this time.

This recipe is structured in consciousness. It can last one

minute or one day, and reoccurs whenever you are fully engaged in action without distraction. The thought that "life is what happens to you while you're busy making other plans" has been attributed to three people, one being John Lennon in his song "Beautiful Boy (Darling Boy)." Hang out with Just Hangin' to make sure you don't miss out on your own life. Let the ease of attention and full participation in the present — that nothingness — be everything.

Deep Impressions

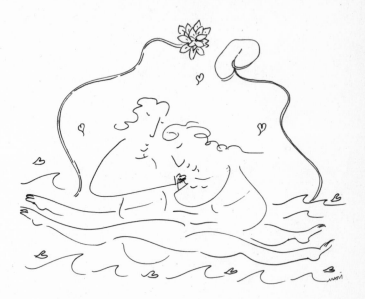

Sometimes the littlest things make the biggest difference.

28. P.S. I Love You

Anything that is written to please a loved one is treasured.

— Rick Eisenberg

- ❦ Attitude of gratitude
- ❦ 1 stockpile of stationery, cards, and Post-it™ notes
- ❦ Ample supply of colored pens
- ❦ 2 e-mail addresses (if available)
- ❦ Internet access for e-cards (if available)
- ❦ 1 banner, sign, or billboard (optional)

*U*se your supply of decorative and humorous cards and blank notes (recipe 2: Love Essentials) to send your partner a thoughtful message whenever the mood hits you. And if lightning doesn't strike, make a vow to yourself to do it anyhow at least once each week. Mark Twain wrote his wife a love letter every day, and they lived in the same house!

If you're online, you can design and send creative e-cards at no charge by going to apple.com and pressing the iCards button. You can also access a large number of free electronic greeting cards on love and romance at passionup.com.

A short note or e-mail expressing gratitude for last night's date or his support during the crisis at work is an excellent way to communicate how much you value your relationship. It shows that even in the midst of your busy day, you are thinking about the one who matters the most. If you want to be dramatic with your feelings, create a banner, special order a message from a sign company, or rent a billboard.

Many women feel that their men rarely think about them when they are at work or away from the house. Men, show them they are wrong!

Sample Serving

I'll never forget peeking out the window one Valentine's Day and seeing the shocked look on Jimmy's face when he arrived home. Stretched across the front of the house was a ten-foot, hot pink laminated banner announcing to him and the entire neighborhood, "Leslie Loves Jimmy." Once inside the house, he followed a trail of notes and chocolate truffles leading him to the bedroom. I could hardly wait for him to open the door.

29. Hidden Delights

The adult version of hide-and-seek.

- ❦ 1 or more cards or 1 pad Post-it™ notes
- ❦ 1 pen or pencil
- ❦ 1 personal computer (if shared)
- ❦ 1 gift that can be hidden
- ❦ 1 ad copy (alternative)

W rite a note or card and put it in an unusual place, but where your partner can't miss it: inside the clothes dryer or tool box, on the car steering wheel or visor, inside a shoe, purse, or briefcase. Post-it™ notes are fun to put all over the house.

If you share a personal computer, you can leave a message on Notepad (PC) or Stickies (Mac), or make up a screen saver with an endearing message that will greet her when she opens it up.

You can take this idea one step further by placing gifts in locations that are unusual yet related to the gift. A box of new clothing might be hidden inside the washing machine, or tickets to a big sporting event can be tucked inside a gym bag. An unusual shade of nail polish could be dropped inside a shoe, or a new paperback might show up under the pillow. (Surprises could also be personally made coupons for simple things you know your partner would appreciate, like "A Drive in the Country" or "Hot Kisses Beneath a Full Moon.")

Another variation is for your loved one to discover your affections in a newsletter, newspaper, or magazine that she reads regularly. A classified or display ad can acknowledge her unique qualities, refer to a tender moment in the relationship, mark a milestone, or propose a tryst. Or you might arrange for a message to be announced on the public address system or flashed on the scoreboard at a sporting event you are both attending. This has become a popular way for sports fans to propose marriage or send an electronic birthday card.

30. Family Ties

They'll love to hear the good news.

- ❧ 1 note or card
- ❧ 1 pen
- ❧ Address of your partner's parents
- ❧ 1 gift or flowers (optional)

*S*end a note of appreciation about your partner to his parents. "Thank you for creating such a wonderful person. (Partner's name) has brought so much joy into my life." Consider including a small gift or flowers.

31. Forever Yours

How do I love thee? Let me count the ways.

— Elizabeth Barrett Browning,
Sonnets from the Portuguese, Sonnet 14

- ❧ Ability to verbalize and record intimate feelings
- ❧ Colored pens or pencils
- ❧ 1 elegant sheet of writing paper
- ❧ 1 handsome frame
- ❧ 1 calligrapher (optional)

What is it about your loved one that really moves you, stirs your being, or makes your heart sing? Let him know how important he is to you by writing down those deepest sentiments in your own words and presenting them to him as a special gift.

Be inspired by love songs and poetry. Your message might include one or more of the following: why your relationship means so much to you; how you feel when you're together; how you felt about her the first time you met, or kissed, or when she said, "I do"; how much you admire his positive attitude or unique qualities; thanks for a wonderful life or for his unconditional love.

Whatever it is you decide to communicate, start by jotting down all of your thoughts on a sheet of paper. Then rewrite your message several times until you are satisfied with it. Captivating songs and poems convey powerful emotions with relatively few words; be precise and concise in your approach. Next, record these private thoughts on a beautiful sheet of paper from a stationery store — or have them transcribed by a calligrapher — and frame it. Choose a handsome frame that your partner might place in a special location, and wrap it up as an elegant gift.

Never underestimate the power of the written word. Your recorded thoughts and feelings may be cherished for many years and be more memorable than an expensive gift that becomes obsolete or no longer is in style.

32. No Excuses

*Distance makes the heart grow fonder,
or yonder. It's up to you.*

- ❧ 10 to 15 minutes each day you're away
- ❧ More than a "Hi, how are you?"
- ❧ 1 to 3 discreetly placed cards or gifts (optional)
- ❧ 2 e-mail addresses with instant messaging (optional)

Whenever you are away from your loved one, at least one phone call daily is a must; always try to share something intimate during each conversation. For added spice, begin the conversation with an offbeat or wild greeting using a foreign accent.

Many couples find it more convenient when they are apart to keep in touch by e-mail. The added separation can actually make you feel more open and bolder in expressing your feelings than you would over the phone. Also, it's often easier to be more reflective and poetic when you communicate your thoughts in writing, as opposed to leaving a voice mail or playing phone tag. With the growing popularity of instant messaging, you can now do all this in a private real-time dialogue over the Internet.

Another way to reach out and touch your loved one is to combine one or two of the calls or e-mails with a little treat. Either by voice or electronically, direct your partner to a place in the house or apartment where you've left a thoughtful card or gift.

33. Going Public

It's better if they're watching.

- ❧ Opportunity to catch your partner with an audience
- ❧ 1 hot beverage in a special mug
- ❧ Pastry, snacks, reading materials (optional)
- ❧ 1 card with flowers
- ❧ Lunch with tablecloth and candles

Surprise your partner at work during a morning or afternoon break with gourmet coffee or tea served in a commuter, vintage, or theme mug. This simple offering will be remembered long beyond your visit and can be expanded to include a favorite pastry, snacks, or reading materials.

Men, don't be so private with your cards and flowers. Send them to a place where other people can admire them with her (work, a luncheon with the ladies). Let her coworkers know if it's your anniversary; send a Happy Anniversary cake to the office.

Ladies, instead of taking him out to lunch, bring a homemade or catered meal to his workplace. Whip out a tablecloth and candles and join him at the newest hot dining spot in town.

Doyle wanted to make a romantic statement with Katherine, his girlfriend of several months. She was working at the time in a restricted business environment where personal visits were not allowed. Doyle, however, was determined to get through security and catch Katherine by surprise.

Searching for a delivery man's outfit in various thrift stores, he found and bought a UPS shirt and a pair of matching brown pants. Then he secured a clipboard and the necessary UPS materials: shipping box, delivery sheet, and label. On the way to Katherine's office, he bought a bouquet of her favorite flowers and placed them carefully inside the box.

When Doyle arrived at the main reception area of Katherine's workplace, the receptionist said she would sign for the delivery. He looked down to check the notes on his clipboard, and informed her that this particular package required the signature of the recipient. When Katherine came downstairs five minutes later, she was amazed to find Doyle waiting for her, looking and acting so professional in his assumed role. Without breaking his cover, he offered a friendly "hello" along with the UPS box and asked for her signature. After she wrote "Lady Godiva" on the appropriate line, Doyle simply said "thank you" and left.

Katherine received many compliments on both the beautiful flowers and the novel way in which they had arrived. Learning about the true identity of the UPS guy, her astonished co-workers recognized what she kept thinking about all that day and for many days to come: there was someone out there who really cared about her, so much that he personally made a "special delivery."

34. Helping Hand

Kindness in giving creates love.

— Lao-tzu

❧ Ability to recognize when your partner needs help
❧ Willingness to render prompt service with a smile

*D*o something that's outside your job description. Offer to help your partner complete some chores she usually does alone. Your intentions will be appreciated even more when you jump in enthusiastically without being asked.

This simple gesture can turn a mundane job into something romantic. A dear friend of ours, with two children, remarried a very busy doctor. She tells us that one of her greatest turn-ons is watching her husband help her son and daughter with their homework after dinner.

Another friend told us she once asked her husband, "What is the most boring thing you've ever done?" Without hesitating, he said, "I don't know why, but washing the car bores me to tears." She took him by the arm and led him outside. "Great, let's do it together." They had a blast, and now there is one less thing in his life to be bored about.

Consider this wonderful piece of advice from Mike and Jennie, the golden anniversary couple mentioned in recipe 22: The Last Goodbye: "Even if you think you're giving 90 percent in your relationship, you're probably not giving 40 percent of what you should." Try the next recipe as a way of giving even more.

35. Devoted to You

*What do we live for, if it is not to make
life less difficult to each other?*

— George Eliot, *Middlemarch*

❧ Generous amount of time (minimum of 4 hours)
❧ Eagerness to serve unconditionally

Obviously, tiredness and stress are not conducive to romance. If your partner is becoming overwhelmed or exhausted by the demands of work, home, or the kids, it's time for you to take charge and ensure that things don't get out of hand.

First, communicate your intentions, then agree on a day when she can sleep in and relax until early afternoon, or be away from the house for a decent block of time. Assure her that, during that period, you will take care of everything she wants and needs to have done: cooking meals, taking care of the kids, running errands, doing specific household chores — whatever it takes to reduce the pressures and lighten her burden. Later, when you reunite and see how appreciative she is, you will be reminded of how much more fulfilling it often is to give than to receive.

This is a powerful way to show your loved one how much you value her comfort and happiness; it will definitely help to keep romance on track! For a more personal type of devotion that allows you to focus only on your partner's immediate romantic and sexual needs, be sure to use recipe 79: Light My Fire.

Special Deliveries

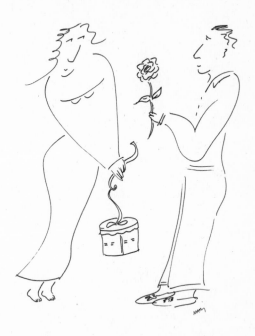

It all comes down to the presentation.

36. Full Throttle

Shift into high gear on gift giving!

- 🐾 1 car
- 🐾 Ability to move unsuspected and undetected
- 🐾 1 or more gifts

The automobile is an American institution associated in memory with scenic road trips, romantic moonlit rides, necking on Lovers' Lane, and perhaps your first time.

Consider letting this keystone of youth serve up more than cherished memories and transportation from point A to point B. Make it a vehicle for surprise gift giving, big or small, anytime.

Imagine how your partner will feel when he slips into the car on a cold morning, and his body sinks into the new sheepskin seat cover. Or the smile on her face when she reaches for those new sunglasses or the necklace hanging from the rearview mirror. The bow on the glove compartment directs him to the invitation to a special concert or rendezvous later that night. And as she starts the car, she discovers on the console a new travel mug with a gift certificate from her favorite coffee bar.

Sample Serving

A single mother, Linda, met a man who seemed like the perfect match for her and her young child. However, she and her Prince Charming had an uncomfortable parting after six weeks because of a misunderstanding. Thoughts of him and what they had shared saddened her during the weeks and months that followed. Almost one year later, she happened to pass him in his car as she drove into the parking lot of a local supermarket. Seeing his face again rekindled the vivid memories of their short time together, and she couldn't help but think about what might have been as she moved up and down the aisles of the store.

When she returned to her car with an armful of groceries, her attention was drawn to a single red rose on the windshield. That simple gesture was the catalyst that brought them together that evening. Within a year they married, and they are still living happily ever after.

37. Value-Added Bouquet

The fragrance goes so much further.

- ❦ 1 bouquet of fresh-cut flowers
- ❦ 1 related or unrelated gift
- ❦ Bountiful imagination

$\mathcal{D}$ouble the pleasure of flowers by adding something extra to the bouquet. It can be a crystal or handblown vase, cutting shears, flower pressing kit, seeds, or an unrelated gift such as handmade chocolates or tickets to the theater.

Many men also enjoy receiving flowers, particularly when they are part of a larger gift idea. If your man doesn't, substitute with a bouquet of balloons. The number of successful combinations are limited only by your sense of imagination.

Sample Serving

When Jimmy buys me fresh flowers, I am often surprised by the creativity behind many of the arrangements. My favorite was a pastel blend of flowers in a beautiful vase. At the top of the bouquet was a solicitation postcard from a dating service I had joined years before. Written over the message that someone wanted to meet me were the words "TAKEN FOR GOOD."

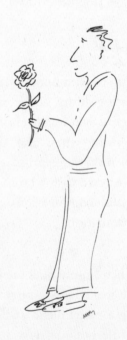

38. Treasure Chest

We store preserves so that sweet fruit
may always be in season.

- 1 memory basket
- Artifacts of love
- Desire to keep on giving

Give your partner a special box or container in which to keep all the love memorabilia you send or share (such as cards, notes, pictures, concert ticket stubs). It can be purchased at a store, or you may want to exercise your artistic talents and make one out of stained glass, metal, or wood.

An inscription on the inside — even something as simple as "From (your initials) to (your partner's initials)" — can be intimately beautiful and remind her of your devotion whenever the time capsule is opened.

39. For Keeps

Create a keepsake that springs from your hands and heart.

- ❦ 1 nickname, term of endearment, or symbol of interest
- ❦ 1 attractive, useful object
- ❦ Ability to emboss, embroider, or customize

C hoose and personalize an object that your loved one can use or wear regularly. Handmade articles, embroidered pillows or clothing, and customized mugs or jewelry offer attractive ways to display a cherished nickname, term of endearment, or a symbol of a special interest. Because of the usability of the item, it will serve as a continual and personal reminder of your affection.

Sample Serving

Leslie once had a boyfriend whose astrological sign was Cancer; he lived on a boat and loved to sail. She surprised him for his birthday with a denim work shirt on the back of which she had embroidered a large crab; on the front pocket was a sailboat with a sunset. She had also replaced all of the buttons with wooden ones that had tiny anchors etched into them. He enjoyed the shirt so much over the next several years that he literally wore it to death.

Tina (of recipe 21: Lighten Up) loves it when Tom refers to her as his "little pea princess." Because she is so physically active and tends to bruise easily, Tom came up with the idea for her nickname from the fairy tale "The Princess and the Pea." For one of Tina's birthdays, Tom visited a jeweler friend and asked him to design a necklace with a small jade pea and gold leaves fastened to a beautiful chain. Tina feels elegant whenever she puts on the necklace. She takes great pleasure in knowing that the jewelry, which radiates Tom's thoughtfulness and sweetness, was custom-made just for her.

40. Satisfaction Guaranteed

The crème de la crème of gift giving!

- ❧ 1 favorite specialty store
- ❧ 1 gift certificate or cash
- ❧ 1 card of appreciation
- ❧ Permission to go for it (giver)
- ❧ Suspension of guilt (receiver)

*D*oes this sound familiar? You've agonized over what gift to buy your loved one because you want it to be just right. When she opens the package, you get a big "thank you" along with a smile and a hug. You rejoice in thinking you have done a good job, until you notice a few days later that the gift has somehow fallen into a black hole, never to be seen again.

Giving a gift that is absolutely sure to please is not as difficult as you might imagine. In fact, it's simple if you listen or observe carefully and familiarize yourself with the kind of gift or store that your partner prefers. Then, take him to that favorite specialty shop — clothing, sporting goods, electronics, antiques, crafts, furniture, jewelry, music, or books

— and present him with a card of appreciation. Inside the card is cash or a gift certificate along with your encouragement for him to spend the entire amount on anything his heart desires.

The amount of your gift does not have to be large — it's the idea of letting your partner buy or splurge on whatever she or he wants, completely on a whim and without feelings of guilt. Just your being there and supporting the choice will add to the meaning of the gift.

For the most dramatic effect, give this marvelous gift at a time when it will not be associated with a birthday or holiday.

41. More to Come

Giving presents is a talent; to know what
a person wants, to know when and how to get it,
to give it lovingly and well.

— Pamela Glenconner,
Edward Wyndhan Tennant: A Memoir

- ❧ Sensitivity to your partner's interests
- ❧ Choice of theme
- ❧ Multiple gifts

A woman told us she was pleased by the gifts her husband gave her during the early years of their marriage — until she discovered that he had been sending his secretary to pick out what she thought his wife would like. The husband learned an important lesson about the care and feeding of romance: The thought does count. What you give is one thing; how you give is everything!

A simple gift that reflects sensitivity to your partner's preferences (recipe 25: The Pleasure List) will be more meaningful than a more expensive one that does not. And a terrific way to increase the joy of receiving is to give him a number of gifts over a period of time that tie into a specific theme. You get to choose the theme; but, remember, be mindful of *his* interests, not your own. As an example, you might consider seasonal seeds for a gardening enthusiast. A wine connoisseur would appreciate a new bottle each month from a choice vineyard. An avid reader would be thrilled to get a first peek at each new hardback release from her favorite author.

Themes provide a good source of future gift ideas and limit the need to use an excuse like, "I have no idea what to get you." When you come up with the right idea, your partner will look forward to what the next theme gift might be. In some cases, his enthusiasm may translate into a desire to start a collection that spans many years; and it may even involve both of you (recipe 7: Partners in Passion).

Sample Serving

Stewart was dating Heather, who liked old folk music. Stewart was also a music lover and happened to be reading a book by David Hajdu called *Positively 4th Street: The Lives and Times of Joan Baez, Bob Dylan, Mimi Baez Fariña, and Richard Fariña*. Heather expressed a keen interest in the book, so Stewart gave it to her as a gift when he finished it.

As the holidays approached, Stewart reflected on Heather's enthusiasm for the things she was learning about in the book. A week before Christmas, he gave her the Joan Baez CD, *Live from Newport*, a recording including Baez's sets from the 1963–1965 Newport Folk Festivals, along with a note that said, "Now that you are reading about this, I thought you might enjoy experiencing it."

Over the next few months, Stewart followed up by surprising Heather with the first recordings of Bob Dylan and Richard and Mimi Fariña, as well as some live Dylan CDs and an old Newport Folk Festival poster. One of his many gestures was particularly touching: a sixties-style sundress and sandals similar to those worn by Joan Baez in photos in the book.

These thoughtful gifts completely won Heather over. She now teaches Stewart to play guitar, and says that whenever she hears an early Dylan or Baez song, she can't help but think of her aspiring student.

42. The Grass Is Greenest . . . Where You Water It

A successful marriage is an edifice that must be rebuilt every day.

— André Maurois

- ❧ Adequate time
- ❧ Focused attention

*E*ach and every day, be sure to do at least one kind thing for your loved one. Even a small, unexpected gesture that comes from the heart will be cherished and serve to nurture love and romance. It's not enough to appreciate your partner in your thoughts; you must give a voice to it. The cumulative effect of these daily overtures will cultivate a beautiful relationship in which you feel blessed to have found each other.

So pay attention to that special person who is closest to you. Open your heart. Speak your love today . . . and tomorrow . . . and the day after.

Breaking Boundaries

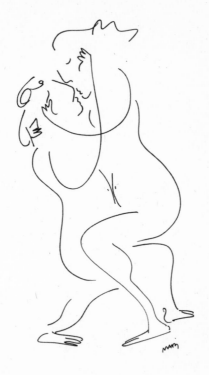

If you hang out in your comfort zone, it becomes your coffin.

— Stan Dale

43. Go Crazy

Love is being stupid together.

— Paul Valéry

- ❦ Lots of enthusiasm
- ❦ Plenty of foolishness
- ❦ Courage to change the ordinary into the extraordinary
- ❦ Eagerness to share the fun (optional)

*S*ome craziness mixed with a touch of giddiness may be just what your relationship needs right now. Get playful with your partner. Have a food, pillow, or tickle fight. Dance around the house or do the dishes together — naked. Eat a candlelit dinner in your walk-in closet. Try on each other's clothes — in the privacy of your home, of course. Go to an all-night supermarket in your pajamas and bathrobe at 2:00 A.M.; you'll fit right in with the other customers!

As with the couple in our sample serving, you may derive a great deal of additional pleasure by encouraging others to get crazy with you.

Kari Ann Gerlach of Love Nest Enterprises (mylovenest.com) decorates bedrooms and baths to create romantic or celebratory settings for clients, many of whom are newlyweds. On one occasion, a California couple decided to expand their wedding night romance to include close family members. They purchased not one but four hotel packages: the Classic package for themselves, the Cupid package (with red satin sheets, red heart garland, and white tulle) for each set of parents, and something extra special for the bride's grandparents from Minnesota.

Because her grandparents were approaching their fiftieth wedding anniversary, the bride wanted to make her wedding night even more memorable for them and asked Kari Ann to give her beloved golden-agers the Animal Attraction package. Imagine their surprise when they opened the door to their room and saw black satin sheets with animal prints and fabric accents, and a big piece of fake fur across the corner of the bed. A number of rather wild conventioneers were staying at the same hotel, and the grandparents were sure they had somehow entered the wrong room. With caution and curiosity, they moved toward the bed to read the note on the pillow. Their mood changed dramatically when they saw, "GRR! Get Wild. Happy Anniversary."

Her grandmother called the next day to thank her and ask if it was okay to take the Animal Attraction package back to Minnesota. "Of course," said Kari Ann, "as long as you use it again on your anniversary next year."

44. Wet Dreams

When it rains, the gods are happy.
— Proverb in India

❧ 1 inviting rain shower or storm
❧ 1 or 2 umbrellas or adequate rain gear

Y ou're safe inside your warm and cozy home while raindrops dance on the rooftop and bounce off the streets and sidewalks. The rain's steady beat and shifts in intensity are a soothing backdrop to cooking and eating, sitting and reading by the fireplace, cuddling as you watch an old movie, or making love.

Rain is often linked with romance, and you may not be taking full advantage of this marvelous gift from nature. The next time a storm rolls in, ask your partner to join you at the front door. Pick up an umbrella or put on some rain gear and boots and go outside together for no reason other than to be touched directly by the rain. Hold hands, kiss, run around, slosh through puddles, or just put your head back and let the water wash against your faces. Be playful;

let yourselves get soaking wet. Once you're over the need to stay dry or look good, you'll begin to feel easier and freer. You may suddenly find ways of having fun in the rain that you never imagined before. And because you are doing it with the one you love, it may have a liberating influence on the relationship itself.

Inside or outside, rain just can't be beat.

Sample Serving

Skip and Debbie (of recipe 23: Do Not Disturb) looked forward to spending the Independence Day weekend in Boston. After they arrived, however, the weather got progressively worse, and the spectacular fireworks display over Boston Harbor had to be canceled because of the heavy storms. Disappointed but determined not to let a little torrential rain spoil their mini-vacation, they headed over to Faneuil Hall, the quaint refurbished marketplace that is full of restaurants, bars, and shops.

Skip and Debbie stopped by an eatery where there was good live music playing; but they couldn't get a seat because the inclement weather had driven so many people indoors. Nevertheless, with one large umbrella covering the two of them, they stood outside in an empty cobblestone courtyard and listened to the band along with the rhythm of the falling rain. One song flowed into another, and then the band started playing "Smoke Gets in Your Eyes." It was one of *their* songs, so Skip did what he had to do: he turned to Debbie and asked her to dance. He held the umbrella steadily above them; they embraced and began to move slowly in step with the beat of the music. The tears of the gods, which earlier that evening had turned them away from the fireworks, now rained down happily on their parade.

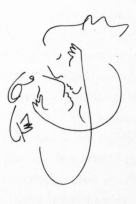

45. Play Date

Our most serious responsibility is not to be serious.

❧ Freedom to go out and let go
❧ 1 large menu of outdoor activities
❧ Willingness to overcome inhibitions
❧ Unlimited smiling and laughter

We marvel at young children. They radiate spontaneity, enthusiasm, and curiosity, and seem to have a boundless reserve of positive energy — the very same qualities we often associate with feelings of falling or being in love. Nevertheless, many of us have grown up believing we have to curb these impulses in order to be effective as adults.

An excellent way for you and your partner to embrace these carefree qualities of youth and love is to periodically schedule a Play Date. What's a Play Date? It's a free pass to go outside on a beautiful day and act like children. Start with physical activities such as running, skipping, jumping, climbing, rolling around, and dancing. Do some of the things that remind you of your own childhood experiences:

kicking puddles after a rainstorm; burying yourself beneath a pile of fallen leaves; finger painting, drawing in the dirt, or making mud pies; going to a playground and using all the equipment; playing games like tag or hide-and-seek; flying a kite; playing ball; having a water pistol fight; lying on your backs on soft green grass and gazing at passing clouds. The possibilities are limited only by your imagination. If you want some additional ideas, observe the children around you and do what they do. And don't forget about water slide and amusement parks, carnivals, and zoos. Those places are kids' heaven.

There are no rules about which activities you should choose, but this recipe produces best results when you encourage each other to try the very things you feel the most inhibited about doing. Children don't feel guilty or foolish when enjoying themselves and neither should you. Smile and laugh along with them; you'll begin to experience the immense joy that comes from the resurgence of childlike innocence. And be sure your Play Date includes a visit to the local ice cream parlor. It is one of the few places on earth where everyone is always happy.

Be advised: the effects of Play Date can be contagious. You may be walking in a crowd when you find yourself giving into the impulse to pull your loved one toward you for a passionate hug and kiss (recipe 1: Hot Lips). Or you might start singing or dancing together for no apparent reason while shopping or dining. Or both of you may call in late for work and start the morning with a long stroll through the park (recipe 3: Kick the Habit). It is a wonderful feeling to be in touch with your childlike nature while you are busy being an adult. Remember, couples that play together stay together.

46. Befriending Your Fear

How bold one gets when one is sure of being loved.

— Sigmund Freud

❦ Clarity of desire
❦ Courage to confront your demons

Almost everyone struggles with an unfulfilled dream or a broken promise of youth. Often it is fear, rather than lack of opportunity, that keeps us away from the road not taken.

Helping your partner overcome fear and actualize a life-long desire can be one of the greatest acts of love. It not only opens the door to a brighter future, but also makes you a richer person for having enriched the life of another. When you encourage him to pursue his dreams against any odds, he will be touched by your unconditional support throughout the process.

Sample Serving

Rick is a talented writer and musician living in New York City. Several years ago, he confided in his girlfriend, Connie, that he had always wanted to be an entertainer, but felt he wasn't a very good singer. Connie had been involved in the performing arts and listened patiently without accepting or rejecting Rick's assumptions. The next day, however, she took action: she went to his apartment, got comfortable on the couch, and asked him to start singing for her.

At first, Rick felt self-conscious and made some mistakes as he performed for his private audience of one. Connie's positive responses and suggestions, though, awakened Rick to the possibility that he might have something to offer after all. In his own words, Rick said the experience "made me feel like a singer." As a result of Connie's coaching and the growth in his confidence over the next several months, Rick did fulfill one of his musical dreams when he auditioned and was hired to sing and play piano every Friday and Saturday night at an Upper West Side restaurant. He never again doubted his ability to sing.

47. Finger Food

*A delicious way to have more
than just time on your hands.*

- ❦ 4 clean hands
- ❦ 2 adventurous spirits
- ❦ 1 restaurant
- ❦ Home sweet home (alternative)

*H*ere's a recipe to generate more intimacy with your partner and your food. Either tell him your intentions in advance, or let them unfold gracefully along with your napkin.

Choose a restaurant that has a diverse menu. After you place your order, ask the waiter to please remove the silverware. Once the food arrives, begin to feed each other the entire meal with your fingers! You're probably going to attract some attention, but it's unlikely that anyone will ask you to stop or to leave. People around you will tend to be curious or fascinated. And who knows? — your carefree behavior may inspire other couples to lighten up and join in.

If you are shy by nature or feel inhibited, try Finger

Food first in the privacy of your home, then step up to a restaurant (like a fried food hangout) where the clientele already have their elbows on the table and eat primarily with their hands. As an alternative, you may want to visit an Indian, Ethiopian, or Middle Eastern restaurant, where eating with the hands is acceptable. Many foreign cultures eat without utensils; delicious breads are often used to facilitate the experience. (Etiquette tip: In the South of India, where they favor soupy curries, juices running down as far as the elbow is considered a bit low class!)

Finger Food is a unique way of using romance to relax, laugh, and create special memories. You'll enjoy the food's textures and tastes more directly, just like you did as a child. And finger feeding can arouse the sensual touching and giddiness you both felt when you first started dating. Once you're hooked, you and your partner will want to do this more often, particularly when you are cooking and eating alone at home. It can serve as marvelous foreplay.

Sample Serving

The most fun we've ever had with this recipe was at the Cajun Crawfish Hut in Long Beach, Mississippi. It is a superb, informal restaurant on the Gulf Coast featuring boiled seafood in one-, two-, and three-pound servings. The owner, Bubba, and his family members are never offended by how you eat or the mess you make. To make their point, every table has a roll of paper towels in place of napkins, and regular customers are encouraged to bring an extra shirt!

48. Going for Broke

*I have enough money to last me the rest
of my life, unless I buy something.*

— Jackie Mason

I've got all the money I'll ever need if I die by four o'clock.

— Henny Youngman

- ❧ 1 day together
- ❧ Empty pockets and purses
- ❧ Ability to control the desire to spend
- ❧ Joy in exercising your creativity

*H*ere's a recipe that surprises a lot of people: Spend one day together without spending any money whatsoever. Do what you might normally do, but avoid using cash or credit cards for any purchases, including food. A day of financial fasting will do both of you a lot of good beyond saving money. You'll discover that you've probably been wasting money on frivolous or unnecessary purchases as you examine the impulses for spending that arise. But, more importantly, you'll find that you don't have to spend *any* money to have a great time.

Your happiness, as individuals and as a couple, depends much more on your creativity than on what's in your wallet or purse. Without money to spend, you can cook together at home or ask close friends or relatives to cook a meal for you. They'll be fascinated with your reason for inviting yourselves over! Or you can play cards or sports, make love, go window-shopping, or take a long drive — if there's enough gas in the car.

A fun day of Going for Broke will remind both you and your partner that many of life's experiences may be enhanced by money, but your happiness does not depend on it. Your greatest lesson in romance is that you don't have to spend a lot of money to express your love. True, money can be helpful; but it alone can never substitute for creativity and kindness.

49. Pushing the Envelope

Don't play for safety. It's the most
dangerous thing in the world.

— Hugh Walpole

❦ Ability to stretch in new directions
❦ Mutual respect and support

*T*he word *romance* was used originally to describe a
medieval narrative depicting heroic or marvelous achieve-
ments, such as those found in the tales of King Arthur and
the Knights of the Round Table. Today, it is still this sense
of excitement and adventure that makes romance so important to us, something we never seem to tire of.

As your relationship evolves, be sure to engage in activities with your mate that challenge both of you and require
you to develop new resources and talents. Though it may be
appropriate for certain couples, you don't have to parachute
out of an airplane or risk your lives climbing the world's
tallest mountains; but your choices should require you to
stretch the limits of your experience and enable you to learn

something new or improve some aspect of your life. You might consider taking a weekend seminar together on communications, relationships, or human sexuality. If you both have two left feet, signing up for ballroom dancing lessons might be helpful (see recipe 8: Poetry in Motion). For some exhilarating outdoor adventure without excessive risk, there are numerous activities such as jogging, mountain biking, rock climbing, ballooning, scuba diving, and river rafting. Of course, a major life decision like starting or expanding your family, moving overseas, or starting a home-based business can be a powerful catalyst for growth.

Pushing the Envelope opens new vistas. The more you push — without creating overload, of course — the better you will feel about yourselves and your capabilities. Life is always fascinating, full of wonder and positive expectation. Because you are sharing the experience and supporting each other every step of the way, it can be a very romantic adventure. Let the advice of McDonald's founder Ray Kroc be your guide to a fulfilling life: when you're green, you grow; when you're ripe, you rot.

The Write Stuff

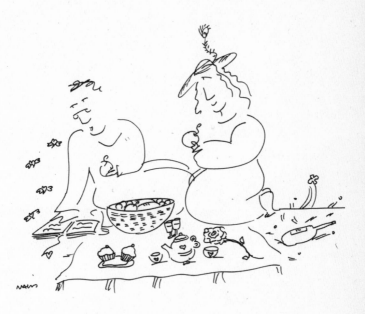

What creative writers can tell us about love and romance.

50. Tropical Getaway

Contributed by Michael Webb,
bestselling author, *The RoMANtic's Guide;*
founder, TheRomantic.com

*A*h! A tropical rain forest! With its beautiful flowers, singing birds, and splashing waterfall you have an instant romantic adventure. No, I'm not going to tell you about a recent trip to some exotic country. Here is how you can have an enchanting rain forest in your own home.

It's so simple I am amazed I didn't think of it earlier. Fill your bathroom with as many plants as you can (no cactus, please). Bring in your music box and play your tape or CD of bird songs or tropical music — even Caribbean music would create the right atmosphere. With some duct tape and a clean dustpan you can easily transform your showerhead into a waterfall.

If you want to go all out, replace your regular lightbulbs with colored ones; blue and green would be a good choice to set the mood. Bring in some candles with scents such as coconut, pineapple, and mango.

Now the next time your loved one needs a getaway but you don't have the time or the money, you can wash away stress and fatigue with a tropical waterfall. It's a lot more creative than your average bubble bath with candles around the tub. Not only will your partner thank you, but also your plants will enjoy the extra special treatment.

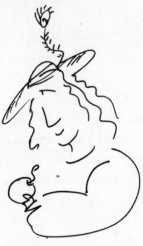

51. My Favorite

Contributed by Buddy Winston,
comedian, former staff writer,
The Tonight Show with Jay Leno

*C*ouples are often advised to learn how to listen to each other. I have found that paying attention to anything that is prefaced with the words "my favorite" is a perfect place to start. I took my girlfriend on a weekend escape to Santa Cruz, California. As we drove through Big Sur, she pointed out the Post Ranch Inn, which she had once told me was her favorite hotel in the world.

I made a U-turn and said I would like to check the place out. She claimed the inn would not allow us to enter without a reservation. When I pulled up to the gate, I asked the security guard if there were any rooms available. He claimed there were none and he could not let us drive in without one. As my girlfriend looked at me with her "I told you so" eyes, I told security that I had a reservation and gave my name. As he welcomed and waved us through, my girlfriend suddenly realized I had planned this in advance just to surprise her. Needless to say, that night the Post Ranch Inn became *my* favorite hotel in the world.

52. Sacred Space

Contributed by Julia Loggins,
co-author (with husband, Kenny Loggins),
The Unimaginable Life: Lessons Learned on the Path of Love

*B*ig Sur, California, is one of the places where Kenny and I fell in love. A romantic and rustic small town, it is bordered by the cliffs of the Pacific Ocean to the west and huge forests of redwood trees to the east. For us, escaping to Big Sur has always represented the ability to disappear from the world, from people, phones, and all earthly responsibilities. It is an idyllic spot for setting up camp by a waterfall deep in the woods, and spending the day writing, reading poetry, making love, and sleeping in the sun.

Our dream was to have a cabin there someday, something small and handmade, where we would do all of the above for days on end. Even our wedding was in Big Sur. Then life entered! Between Kenny's three children — then two and a half, seven, and nine — and the births of our two, romantic weekends quickly segued into soccer games, trips to the zoo, and family barbecues. We have read a lot of poetry, though — most of it Dr. Seuss!

Since we've shared our bed with our babies (and it's so cozy, even big kids love morning snuggles there), our "coupleness" began to dissolve, as every dream we had of making a life together came true in spades. Funny how life is! We yearned for our romantic cabin dream, but two or three days away from the babies was too painful for Mama. Our solution? Kenny converted a tiny bedroom in our guesthouse into a "Big Sur love shack" complete with a clawfoot tub and lanterns and candles for lighting. Many nights, the only light is the moon peering in through a skylight over the bed. Our escape is minutes away, and it is our favorite date nightspot.

Sometimes we just talk. There is a lot more on our plate than there was twelve years ago when we fell in love! Whether we laugh, cry, chat about the nuts and bolts of living or what we're feeling deep in our hearts, we always reconnect. A dear friend gave us a plaque that reads, "The best thing a father can do for his children is love their mother." Our Sacred Space gives us the opportunity to do just that.

53. For a Sleepless Night

Contributed by Jeff Arch,
screenwriter, *Sleepless in Seattle*

Rather than rely on me, try a recipe that my wife would say is very romantic. It's something almost every guy can do, although maybe not at first. On the plus side, it costs no money, requires no elaborate planning, and you don't even have to leave the house to do it. And — maybe best of all, for those who tend to freeze up creatively — a girl already thought of this. So in most situations, it's a good bet that it'll hit home.

It works best at night, and even better after she has had a really rough day — if so, she might have left a few subtle clues around. Here it is then, in a simple step-by-step process that almost any guy — if he's willing to tough it out — should be able to follow:

1. Rub her feet.
2. Don't think of it as foreplay.
3. Just rub her feet.

4. For as long as she wants.
5. Remember Step #2.
6. And then go to sleep holding her.

For a lot of guys, this simple act is more challenging than carving a new face into Mount Rushmore while holding a bucket of live eels in each hand. Most women realize this. And if they don't, don't hold it against them. Just rub their feet, and if you possibly can, restrain yourself. There will definitely be a payoff down the road somewhere.

In closing, I just want to remind every guy out there that this might not make a whole lot of sense. All I'm saying is, it came to me from a really good authority.

P.S. If *she* thinks of it as foreplay, you're good to go.

54. For Women Only
What Guys Think Is Romantic

Contributed by Jeff Arch,
screenwriter, *Sleepless in Seattle*

A lot of women know that what guys like most is sports. Unfortunately, for many of you, this is as far as it goes. You want to join your man in his world — or at least visit him there — but you feel intimidated by your lack of Guy Sports Knowledge (GSN).

Now, thanks to this short and easy guide, almost any woman can "cross over" into GSN Territory and not be too sorry that she did. All you'll need to know is at least one key phrase to say during the contest (it might be a "game" and it might be a "match"), and if you practice being casual about it and pick the right moment, your stock could soar like the space shuttle, and you could find yourself achieving romance in almost no time at all — or faster!

A warning, though: just in case you doubt the potential of what you are about to learn, I'll tell you a quick story. I was walking to a restaurant with my friend Elliott, who I've known all my life. With us was a girl we'll call "Laurel," because that was her name. I had only known Laurel for a few months, and this was the first time Elliott had met her.

During this walk, which was less than a block and a half, Laurel said something that I don't remember exactly but it clearly contained the phrase "San Francisco Giants."

Immediately — immediately — Elliott turned to me and encouraged me in the strongest available terms that I should marry her. If possible, before we even got to the restaurant.

Laurel and I each married different people, and everything's fine all around. All I'm telling you is that this happened over twenty years ago and I still remember the look on Elliott's face when Laurel mentioned the Giants. It was the look people get in the movies when suddenly they hear music.

Okay? So do not — I repeat, DO NOT — underestimate the power of what I am about to tell you.

I've broken the list down into three categories: first, whether the contest he's watching is a game, match, or event; second, how to tell which sport it is that's being played; and finally, a carefully selected quote that goes with the sport and is guaranteed to make your guy drop his Doritos™ right on the spot.

Baseball
Type of contest: Game
How to recognize: There will be men on the field scratching their private parts.
Thing to say: "Name me one time — *one time* — when the Red Sox made a good trade."

Football

Type of contest: Game

How to recognize: There will be men scratching their private parts AND butting their heads together ferociously. These men will be on the same team.

Thing to say: "They get to the Red Zone, and they choke. Is that the story of this team, or what?"

Basketball

Type of contest: Game

How to recognize: There will be men with seven-figure sneaker deals, yet watch them miss this foul shot. Also, Jack Nicholson might be there.

Thing to say: "I can't believe these guys — they're deadly from the perimeter AND in the paint!"

Ice Hockey

Type of contest: Game

How to recognize: There will be men pulling each others' shirts off so they can hold their heads in place and punch them really hard.

Thing to say: "My grandmother could have blocked that shot!"

Tennis

Type of contest: Match

How to recognize: Very solemn line judges who have obviously been bribed, or they wouldn't have just made that call.

Thing to say: "I taped the Kournikova match for you."
(Caution: he may propose on the spot. Be prepared.)

Golf
Type of contest: Match. Endless match
How to recognize: Nobody will be scratching their private parts. Nobody will be doing anything. They're all dead.
Thing to say: "Is he still alive?"

The Olympics
Type of contest: Event
How to recognize: More commercials than ants at a picnic, followed by warmhearted personal profiles about a fifteen-year-old gymnast who has already had thirty-six knee operations, with the occasional televised glimpse of a sport going on. Also, teams from other countries are involved. If you watch carefully, you might actually spot one. But only if we beat them.
Thing to say: "You know, I almost hate to say it but I sort of miss the East Germans."

Well, there you have it. It takes practice and dedication, but I promise it will be time well spent. And if you get frustrated, try to remember — it's not that guys aren't romantic. We're just idiots. But we *can* be reached.

55. Bella Luna

Contributed by Cynthia Daddona,
author of *Diary of a Modern Day Goddess* and inspirational
speaker (www.moderndaygoddess.com)

Whenever I see a full moon, I think of the romantic comedy *Moonstruck* and the song lyrics, "When the moon hits your eye, like a big pizza pie, that's *amore*." I also remember my Italian grandfather, who, at age ninety-one, would burst into song with *"O sole mio"* at the dinner table because he felt loved or was so happy looking at the full, *bella luna* (beautiful moon).

The full moon is a continual reminder of the abundance we are capable of feeling in our hearts, and it can be a signal to strengthen the connection with both your partner and your inner spirit of love and lightheartedness. A touch of creativity, a full-moon night, a candle, a few pieces of handmade or keepsake paper, colored pens, an ornate box, and some music such as the *Moonstruck* soundtrack or Van Morrison's "Moon Dance" are the only requirements. Or, create an intimate Italian feeling with the music of Pavarotti or Andrea Bocelli and by feeding each other grapes and other fresh fruit.

On the night of the full moon, take your loved one to a secluded setting with an unobstructed view of the heavens. Make yourselves comfortable, light a candle, and write down on one sheet of paper the qualities you appreciate about each other. Then, on separate sheets, write down a wish for your mate's happiness and a desire you would like to manifest as a couple (such as more quiet time, a vacation, having a baby). Read these out loud, and express gratitude for the difference you have made in each other's life. Then put on your selection of music and dance beneath the moonlight.

Personally, I like to include two handmade wreaths in my ceremonies so that I can crown myself and my loved one. These can be made easily with supplies from a craft shop. You will need several strands of silk ivy, silk flowers, and some floral wire. Use these ingredients to form the wreaths. For the male (Caesar) version use only ivy. The female version (Aphrodite) can be a combination of ivy and flowers. It's also fun to keep these as a surprise.

When the evening is over, you will still have all those tender acknowledgments and dreams for the future recorded on paper. Place them in the ornate box so you can reflect on them periodically. Writing down your wishes and releasing them to the universe is a powerful ritual that creates the possibility for miracles. Don't be surprised if you find yourselves looking forward to monthly reunions, when you can marvel simultaneously at your love and the moon. *Bella luna!*

56. Down in Front

Contributed by Eric Eisenberg,
playwright, *The Arrangement*

*T*here is something about witnessing a great singer up close that can transport you and your mate to a thrilling, romantic plane neither of you may have quite experienced before. The sound of a beautiful and passionate human voice, pulsating with rich, lustrous tone through a darkened, hushed arena, has provided joy and ecstasy to millions of ears and hearts for centuries — and continues to do so in auditoriums and opera houses around the world today.

My girlfriend and I shared such an experience when we attended, from a close-up box, a performance of Luciano Pavarotti singing in the great Puccini opera, *Tosca*, at New York's Metropolitan Opera House. Although we had seen Pavarotti many times on television and on video, and had even seen him sing live from distant seats at the Met, we had never seen him this close — now less than twenty feet away. The effect, visually and audibly, was astonishing. Not only was the great tenor's wide range of facial expressions vividly clear, but also his sweet, romantic, bell-like tones were heard as if they sang inside our own hearts. It was as if Luciano had invited us to a private recital and was pouring all the world's yearning for love into each fervent note.

Through three and a half hours of musical bliss, we shared an experience so joyous and powerful, neither of us could have comprehended or anticipated it beforehand. It was so powerful, in fact, that it brought us closer together in a way only truly great — and greatly truthful — music can.

So the next time you see that your favorite singer — whoever it may be — is coming to town . . . go! Treat yourself and your loved one to the best seats you can afford. You'll find the investment will provide dividends to the soul that will last for a very long time.

57. Spontaneity Rules

Contributed by Cherie Carter-Scott, Ph.D.,
bestselling author, *If Love Is a Game, These Are the Rules*

*O*ne of the greatest tragedies is to ignore a perfectly healthy and happy relationship and let it slowly slide into complacency. It is terribly important to keep the spark of love alive and glowing. One of the best ways to do this is through spontaneity. Being spontaneous means that you become like children who surprise each other with treats, special events, and just plain fun.

One day my husband, Michael, said, "This Friday you and I are going away somewhere. Be at the front door at 4:00 P.M. I'll take care of packing whatever you need; your only job is to show up on time." I hardly knew what to think. It wasn't my birthday, our anniversary, or Valentine's Day. It wasn't a national holiday or a three-day weekend, and as far as I knew, we weren't celebrating anything. He refused to tell me any more, so I spent the rest of the week wondering about the destination, the logistics, the climate;

I wondered whether he could really pack for me. By mid-week, I was tingling with excitement and suspense.

On Friday, I was ready at the front door, on time. We got into the car and drove to Burbank Airport. As he ushered me toward the gate marked Las Vegas, I knew: he had planned a weekend getaway! After we checked into our hotel, he escorted me blindfolded through the lobby. People were really curious, but stranger things happen in Vegas. He led me to the showroom, where we had front row seats to see my favorite comedienne. This is one of my most fun and delightful memories. Thinking of it still makes me feel special and brings a smile to my face. Create pleasant spontaneous surprises to celebrate the two of you!

Chez Shangri-la

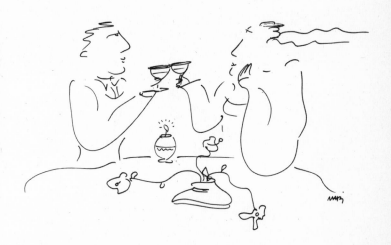

Peace and rest at length have come
All the day's long toil is past,
And each heart is whispering, "Home,
Home at last."

— Thomas Hood, "Home at Last"

58. French Bath

The perfect combination of privacy, togetherness,
mind-body rejuvenation, and uninterrupted pleasure.

- ❦ 1 hour minimum to immerse
- ❦ 1 hot bath with all the trimmings
- ❦ Wine or champagne, fresh fruit,
  poetry (recommended)
- ❦ 1 gift-wrapped bath accessory (recommended)
- ❦ Sea mud or clay (optional)
- ❦ 2 terry cloth robes (optional)

*T*he early Greeks and Romans popularized communal
bathing as part of their daily routine, and the Turks added
the steam; but it wasn't until the dawn of the Renaissance
that couples began to enjoy private baths with hot water. We
can thank the French for replacing the round tub with a
longer, oval-shaped design; and that, coupled with the availability of clean, hot, soothing water, is what allows us in
today's world to lie back and really luxuriate.

Don't overlook this sensuous setting for romance.
Taking a bath together can take on special meaning with a

few small gestures: clear away any bathroom clutter and replace it with flowers and candles; add bubbles, colognes, essential oils, or herbs and teas to the water; introduce exotic soaps; listen to your favorite music; and have your wine or champagne glasses and fresh fruit within easy reach. You might want to include a gift-wrapped bath accessory like a massager brush, heart-shaped loofah sponge, or bath tray. Painting each other's face and neck with sea mud or clay adds a delightful and playful activity and accentuates the therapeutic benefits of the experience. For a literary touch, take turns reading poetry to each other or catch up on your favorite reading material.

Allow for at least an hour to get the most out of this one. Let your cares rise gently and evaporate like the steam. Afterward, feeling warm and relaxed, you may want to wrap yourselves up in terry cloth bathrobes and cuddle in front of a fire or in another favorite spot. We've found this to be an ideal time for Easy Listening (recipe 20) and foot massages.

59. Homecoming

*There is a special place in life where all fatigue
dissolves and the spirit is soothed.*

- Empathy for your partner's burden
- 1 settled home environment
- Help from the kids (if necessary)
- 1 inviting bath
- 1 massage (optional)
- 1 or more gifts (optional)

Remember the family TV shows from the fifties? The cheerful housewife welcomed her tired husband home each evening with the newspaper, his slippers, and a relaxing drink. He usually sat in front of the fire with a friendly dog at his side.

The current workforce often includes both parents. Neither one has the energy for the welcome-home pampering of the good old days. However, if you notice that your loved one is approaching burnout, don't stand around and hope for the best — intervene. Let your home serve the purpose for which it was intended; turn it into a sanctuary of joy and relief.

Take care of all important household responsibilities so he won't have to worry about anything when he walks through the door. Provide a gentle transition from the working grind by avoiding negative talk about bills, car problems, or the hassles of your day. Have dinner ready or order it in. If you have children, enlist their help in waiting on him, hand and foot.

Be sure to prepare him a long hot bath, and follow it with a neck-and-shoulder or full-body massage, if possible. You may also want to include a few small gifts. Home coming conveys a significant message: you notice your partner needs some extra-special attention and you'll go the extra mile to give it to him.

Sample Serving

Betsy works long hours during budget time at her job. One evening as she dragged herself up the front walkway at eight o'clock, she was surprised to see her husband, John, standing by the front door. "Drop everything — your books, folders, and your purse — and come with me right now," he insisted. Betsy followed him into the bathroom, where she received her next instruction, "Enjoy yourself." As he walked out and closed the door, John noticed tears welling up in his wife's eyes.

Betsy took a few moments to appreciate all that John had done: the room glowed in candlelight; classical music filled the air; a bath had been drawn; an open bottle of her favorite wine and a glass sat within reach of the tub. Betsy undressed quickly and slipped into the inviting hot water. As each minute passed, she could feel the stresses from the last few weeks at work ease out of her body. The combination of soothing water, cool wine, and relaxing music acted as a tonic that revitalized her spirit.

Half an hour later, Betsy wrapped herself in a cozy bathrobe and went out to the living room, where John awaited her. As they sat by the fire and enjoyed a romantic husband-made dinner, she reflected on how much John's level of effort meant to her that night. As a result of his thoughtful gestures, Betsy felt a genuine renewal in their love and was prepared to face three more weeks of budget crunch.

60. Foreign Affair

Feast on each other and your love will feed on itself.

- ❦ Exotic food
- ❦ Ethnic costume
- ❦ Romantic music
- ❦ Pleasing environment

*T*urn your home into the hottest dining spot in town. Start with your own menu or order a meal for two from a caterer or restaurant specializing in exotic foods. Add the appropriate dress, music, and ambience to draw out the full flavor. Allow this concoction to simmer for an hour or two and your partner will really be salivating.

Sample Serving

Anna is a sensational gourmet cook. One evening her boyfriend, Peter, walked through the front door and found himself transported to India. He was captivated by the aroma of incense and foreign spices, and began to relax immediately to the sitar music of Ravi Shankar. His girlfriend, moving quietly around the living room in her turquoise and gold sari, had covered the coffee table with batik cloths and arranged it with candles and a variety of chutneys. Anna invited Peter to join her on the floor, where they lounged on cushions and ate samosas, curries, saffron rice, and breads with their fingers. Within minutes, he felt as though he had joined her on an exotic journey and left his troubles behind. After dinner, Peter sipped mango *lassi* as Anna introduced him to the *Kama Sutra*.

61. Endless Shower

The perfect way to start the day.

- A little more time than usual
- 1 exotic shampoo, exfoliating scrub, and shower gel
- 1 to 2 hot coffees or teas
- 2 to 4 breakfast pastries and fruit
- 2 warmed-up, perfumed bath towels

Ask your partner to take a nice long, hot shower when neither one of you is rushed for time. You may want to stock up beforehand with exotic shower products: a kiwi-melon shampoo, rosemary-mint salt scrub, and mango shower gel are likely to invigorate the appetite. Bring in coffee or tea with scones, bagels or muffins, and tropical fruit, and await your partner with two bath towels, just heated in the dryer and sprayed with perfume or essential oil (recipe 6: Two Scents' Worth).

62. Royal Treatments

True nurturing starts in one direction
and quickly goes both ways.

- Generous amount of private time
- 1 giver and 1 receiver
- 2 to 3 homemade treatments
- Plenty of water and towels
- Assorted oils, lotions, and potions (as needed)
- A selection of favorite foods, flowers, candles, music
- Massage classes (optional)

Convert your home into a private day spa where the options are many and the treatments are free. The possibilities for your partner's pleasure will be a function of your creativity combined with your skills. It can be as simple or as extravagant as you desire, a prelude to a date or a full day of luxury. When considering the treatments to offer your "spa guest," you can get inspiration online or visit a professional spa and look at a list of its services.

To create an inviting spa atmosphere, preparation is critical. Be sure you have all the necessary ingredients ready beforehand. These may include lotions, oils, towels, bubble bath, hair and body treatments, as well as favorite foods, flowers, candles, and soothing music. Also, plan ahead to eliminate potential distractions that might interfere with your privacy. Turn off phones and turn on voice mail: let callers know you are in a very important meeting and cannot be disturbed.

It's important that partners maintain their respective roles as giver and receiver throughout the spa activities. The touch of the giver transfers loving energy to the receiver, whose glowing satisfaction is reflected back to the provider of her pleasure. This gentle cycle of giving and receiving/receiving and giving has a soothing and profound healing influence on each person. Should you try to assume both roles in one day, the giver may begin to anticipate his time to receive and be distracted from giving full attention to his loved one, and the receiver may not be able to fully relax if she has to think about how and when to reciprocate.

This recipe can be a surprise treat for your partner, or it can be planned jointly with the two of you trading places on a follow-up occasion. Either way, it's like taking a mini-vacation that is emotionally energizing. If this is something you decide to do on a regular basis, the experience will be greatly enhanced if you take a massage class together.

For Cupid's arrow to soar, it must first be drawn back far on the bow. Think of Royal Treatments as a special time and place to relax, touch, fully appreciate and enjoy each other's bodies and presence, and revitalize your relationship for the next stage of your romantic journey.

Sample Serving

One of our Italian friends, Chiara, first told us about this recipe, which she likes to put into action with her husband, Alex, whenever they feel a need to replenish their reserves. The following is an example of what Chiara does when she initiates the day's activities:

As part of preparation, she arranges for her son to have an overnight with one of his best friends, which creates special time for him as well; and she makes sure he will not be coming back to the house before midafternoon, at the earliest.

Chiara and Alex like to start their day with gentle caresses. When they are ready to get out of bed, she prepares a light breakfast of toast or almond croissants with coffee or tea. It is followed by some light exercise — either walking or lovemaking. Then she begins the first treatment, a full-body massage. Alex welcomes the extra attention she gives to his hands and feet. The lighting is low, scented candles fill the room with a calming fragrance, and the choice of music adds to the relaxation. After the massage, Chiara prepares a bath for Alex. He enjoys the way she gently bathes him while his face tingles beneath a purifying masque. She scrubs his back and rubs a hair treatment into his scalp. When the in-bath treatments are finished, Chiara adds hot water and lets her fully relaxed lover soak in silence as she prepares a fabulous brunch. They often eat in the nude and always leave the dishes until the next day.

Chiara has given Alex a timely gift; she is uplifted and gratified by the many kudos she receives and how much lighter he feels as a result of her touch. She also knows how joyfully he will assume the role of giver on the next occasion.

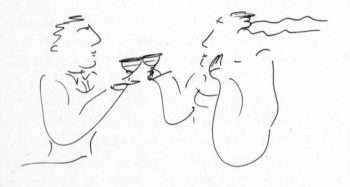

A Breath of Fresh Air

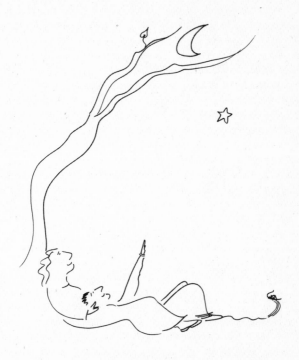

*Another glorious day, the air as delicious
to the lungs as nectar to the tongue.*

— John Muir, *My First Summer in the Sierra*

63. Walk and Talk

Steal your partner away for the pause that refreshes.

- 2 pairs of walking shoes or sneakers
- Active listening
- Eagerness to communicate feelings
- Warm clothing (as needed)

Remember what it was like when you first fell in love and wanted to spend every possible minute with your partner, go everywhere with her, and listen to everything she had to say? Romance and communication are intertwined; intense feelings of love will warm or cool depending on how much time and attention you and your partner are able to give each other.

Maintaining strong and frequent communication to support romance is as easy as putting one foot in front of the other for at least twenty to thirty minutes daily. Be sure to include daily walks together as part of your schedules; they require little or no planning and can be done almost anywhere.

Don't let the elements deter you. A walk in the rain or falling snow can be as romantic as a stroll beneath a full moon. You can vary it by driving to a different neighborhood or hiking trail and starting from there, or by picking unusual times. Predawn and postmidnight sojourns can offer wide differences in experience.

Full and complete attention means just that: no cell phones or pagers allowed!

Sample Serving

A friend of ours is an ordained minister in New Jersey. He advises the couples he marries to take a walk together every day. He and his wife have rigorously followed that advice during their twenty-three-year marriage and call it the secret of their success as a couple. For them, the walk creates a relaxed setting to share or vent "stuff" that might not get out otherwise; they found it far superior — and so may you — to sitting and talking at home, where distractions can occur. And even if there's nothing in particular to relate, it's a great way to exercise and take in some fresh air.

64. Starry-eyed

The stars awaken a certain reverence, because though always present, they are inaccessible.

— Ralph Waldo Emerson

- ❧ Awareness of celestial events
- ❧ 1 clear night
- ❧ 4 eyes wide open
- ❧ 1 to 2 flashlights
- ❧ Warm clothing and beverage (as needed)
- ❧ Pillows, blankets, snacks (optional)

*T*he endless canopy of the night sky is an open invitation to romance, rich in variety and intrigue. It's just outside your door and it's free. Don't take the heavens for granted; plan an evening out with your partner that makes celestial light the center of attention!

You don't have to be an astronomer to appreciate the silent beauty of the constellations or the majesty of a full moon. And there are once-in-a-lifetime occurrences — eclipses, meteor showers, comets — that can be viewed with the naked eye and treasured for a lifetime. Local and national media, particularly the Weather Channel, will give you a heads up on approaching events. For planning purposes, information on more distant phenomena can be accessed over the Internet. Check out these informative and user-friendly websites:

- www.almanac.com/details/moondays.html for the names and dates of all full moons for the next five years
- www.stardate.org/nightsky/ for planet viewing and constellation guides, and a schedule of upcoming comets or meteor showers
- www.usno.navy.mil/ for just about everything related to celestial observing

Sample Serving

It was mid-November 2001, and Santa Barbara was buzzing in anticipation of a weekend of stargazing. That year's Leonid meteor shower was expected to be one of the most dramatic and breathtaking celestial spectacles ever, and many people were gearing up for all-nighters to watch it.

Sadly, Amy didn't feel up to it. She and her husband, Tom, an avid hiker, were early-to-bed/early-to-risers, and raising two small children was so exhausting that missing a night's sleep, even for the meteor showers, seemed impossible.

The more Tom thought about it, though, the more he was determined to give Amy the gift of the best show in town. After much discussion, she gave in reluctantly, provided Tom made all the arrangements. Tom was thrilled and assured her she would never regret it.

Saturday, the children were happily spending the night with Tom's parents, and Amy was able to take a relaxing bath and go to bed at eight. She was awakened by Tom's soft kisses at midnight. They drove to the nearby mountains and encountered bumper-to-bumper traffic near the summit. Amy was amazed to see so many people driving and milling around at that hour of the night; excitement was definitely in the air.

Tom found a place to park by the side of the road. Holding a flashlight in one hand and carrying a large gear bag with the other, he guided Amy through brush and rocks to an ideal vantage point. It was close to 2:00 A.M., and Amy was feeling alert and happy, as though they were explorers making a big discovery. Tom opened his gear bag and took out blankets, pillows, snacks, and a large thermos of their favorite coffee. Touched by his thoughtfulness and enthusiasm, Amy knew in that moment that she didn't want to be anywhere else.

The couple leaned back and watched the countless meteors streaming across the sky. Periods of silence alternated with intimate conversation and lovemaking until dawn, when the celestial showers were replaced by a magnificent sunrise.

65. Doubles Partners

Love is a game that two can play and both win.

— Eva Gabor

- 🌰 1 new outdoor activity or sport
- 🌰 Leisure time
- 🌰 Lessons (optional)
- 🌰 Staying power

$\mathcal{G}$et yourselves outside for some fun on a regular basis. Decide on an outdoor activity or sport that both of you are enthusiastic about learning and doing on a regular basis: gardening, golf, tennis, softball, swimming, hiking, climbing, biking, camping, plein air drawing or painting, sailing, kayaking, or snorkeling. You may want to hire or barter for the services of an instructor, coach, or guide. Along with the joy of learning new skills together, you get physical gain without pain and will probably meet a lot of people who share similar interests.

Sample Serving

Ken and Katie rented a home on Long Island fifteen years ago. It was a large property with a tennis court and pool, and they decided to rent out one of the extra rooms so they could more easily afford it. As it turned out, the tenant they chose was friendly with a tennis pro, who offered to occupy one of the other rooms in exchange for lessons. Neither Ken nor Katie had ever played tennis, so they decided to take advantage of the opportunity to learn a new sport from their live-in pro.

What started out as a simple diversion and a convenient way to exercise turned into a driving passion. Ken and Katie have since moved to California, where they excel competitively in singles and doubles, and occasionally win tournaments as mixed-doubles partners. Their young children are following in their sneaker-steps, and they have met many of their close friends on the courts.

66. Topless

A car can massage organs which no masseur can reach.

— Jean Cocteau, *Opium*

- 1 hot convertible
- 1 generous friend or rental agency
- Plenty of sun
- Lots of leisure time

If you've been spending too much time inside your mind, home, or office and yearn for an exhilarating outdoor adventure, what could be more romantic than cruising down a scenic highway or meandering along backcountry roads in a convertible? Without telling your mate, borrow one from a friend, or rent it from a local agency. If your budget allows, be sure to try out one of the new hot sports cars.

Once you've got your convertible and a beautiful day, the only thing left to do is enjoy. Feel the sun on your faces and the wind in your hair as you bask in your newfound freedom. Look up and share the thrill experienced by convertible owners: there's nothing between you and the sky. You may have chosen a much-talked-about out-of-town restaurant or a cozy bed-and-breakfast as your destination. Or perhaps you'll want to drive without an agenda, giving yourselves the flexibility to stop and picnic, shop, or check out any number of roadside attractions whenever you feel like it. Whatever your course of action, it will gratify your ego to press the pedal to the metal and catch the envious eyes of those you pass.

67. Nature's Table

The settings are as endless as your imagination.

- 🌿 1 enticing outdoor setting
- 🌿 1 prepacked meal and beverage
- 🌿 Adequate time to enjoy
- 🌿 Portable CD or tape player (optional)

There is something inherently festive and romantic about eating outdoors. It is an open invitation from nature to partner with the weather and break out of typical mealtime routines. A picnic can be as simple as some sandwiches in the park or as elaborate as an alfresco feast that has been carefully planned in advance. Try experimenting with different combinations of recipes and locations. There are numerous cookbooks and websites dedicated entirely to picnicking and barbecuing that have menus and practical information such as ways to keep food fresh and prevent leaks and spills on the way to your destination. There's nothing like soggy sandwiches to spoil the mood of a lovely outing!

The number one rule of a successful picnic: never be in a hurry. Romance does not ripen well under pressure. Better to reschedule than press against the clock. You want to have sufficient time to enjoy your surroundings and do fun things like watch the clouds drift by, daydream together out loud or read poetry to each other, take a walk, or fly a kite.

A picnic is not restricted to daytime in warm weather. Full moon nights supply plenty of light to take in a lovely evening; and even in winter, sitting by a bonfire with sandwiches and a hearty soup or hot chocolate from a thermos will help offset the chill factor.

Sample Serving

Robin and Chris love to pack a picnic basket and drive, with their bicycles, to the nearby wine country. They bike through the beautiful countryside and do tastings at several wineries until they find the perfect vintage to complement the goodies in their basket. Then they retreat to a shady picturesque spot to relax with a leisurely lunch.

Jack and Helen enjoy picnicking on the Sheep's Meadow in New York's Central Park. Since they are both actors, they like to enhance their lunch by reading scenes from the works of their favorite playwrights: Shakespeare, Eugene O'Neill, Tennessee Williams, David Mamet, and Neil Simon. The fun really starts when other theatrical picnickers saunter by and join in. Some of these interlopers have even become theatrical comrades of Jack and Helen and have joined them in off-Broadway productions.

Nicole will never forget the formal picnic arranged by her Scottish boyfriend, Michael. As they lounged on a plaid wool blanket in a mountainous area reminiscent of his beloved Scottish highlands, Michael served the food from antique silver pieces that had belonged to his grandmother onto elegant heirloom china. As Nicole ate delicate cookies and tea for dessert, he read the eighteenth-century poetry of his fellow countryman, Robert Burns.

Kim and Frank look forward to weekends when they can visit their favorite bakery at the crack of dawn and fill their basket with warm-from-the-oven pastries. They also order lattes and head directly to the beach, where they hope to make the first footprints of the day in the sand.

Karen and Larry like to picnic during outings on their jet skis. They love the gentle rocking motion on the water and the feeling of solitude. It offsets the excitement of going at high speeds with so much engine noise.

Our most unusual picnic took place during a guided canoe trip. It began at sunset in the Louisiana swamplands outside of New Orleans. With headlamps to light the way, we caught the attention of numerous alligators as we paddled to a place that, without exaggeration, could be called the "middle of nowhere." Despite a mediocre meal and countless mosquitoes that feasted on us that night for dinner, the experience was surprisingly romantic — maybe because we were crazy enough to do it when Leslie was six months pregnant.

68. Season's Greetings

*Nature never wears a mean appearance. Neither
does the wisest man extort her secret, and lose
his curiosity by finding out all her perfection.*

— Ralph Waldo Emerson, "Nature"

- Eagerness to grow with the flow
- Spring equinox, around March 21
- Summer solstice, around June 21
- Fall equinox, around September 21
- Winter solstice, around December 21

The greatest show on earth is just outside your door.
Nature tends to let you in on some of its deepest secrets during the change of seasons. You and your partner can create unique romantic experiences by going outside together and actively observing and listening to what nature can reveal to you. Notice the subtle and dynamic transformations in plant and animal life that go along with shifts in weather patterns, temperature, and the amount of daily sunlight.

Hold hands as you walk together; take a series of deep

breaths; put your faces into the wind; *feel* the earth beneath your feet as you compress leaves, crunch snow, or walk barefoot on a luscious carpet of grass. As you connect with nature's rhythms, you may begin to develop rituals that honor and celebrate these changes. Then, with the advent of each season, you will have something really special to look forward to: a meaningful interaction with the world's most beautiful entertainer.

Sample Serving

Tom and Janis live on a lake in New Hampshire. They have integrated the beauty and joy of the seasons into their routines throughout the year. They know winter has ended when they hear the first call of the loon, the oldest living species of bird on the planet. The return of the loons to the lake corresponds with the beginning of spring, when Tom and Janis like to hike various terrains on a nearby mountain and visit ecological neighborhoods to monitor how the new season is progressing. A special focus for them is searching for small clusters of the elusive Lady Slipper orchids, which often go for years without blooming.

As summer solstice approaches, their attention turns to life on the lake and their adopted children, the loons, whose eggs are just beginning to hatch. Tom and Janis take dinner in a picnic basket, or food to barbecue on a camping grill, and go out on their pontoon boat to a nature preserve area. There they will float until sunset on many summer evenings, watching in awe as a loon family teaches its chicks to dive, fish, and fly.

The magnificence of fall foliage in New England, which starts to accelerate around the time of the equinox, is something Tom and Janis never take for granted. They try to experience it every way they can — in their boat or car or while hiking into the mountains. One of Tom's favorite activities is to send brilliantly colored leaves in airtight plastic bags to his friends in California, Arizona, and Florida. He says this simple gesture has stirred up so many fond childhood memories among its recipients that he has made it an annual ritual.

The winter solstice is a time of thanksgiving for Tom and Janis. They join their lake neighbors around a bonfire on a beach for an evening of socializing and singing Christmas carols. There will be ice skating on the lake if it has frozen. Everyone helps trim a Christmas tree by hanging gloves and mittens from home that will later be donated to a local charity. The feeling of community is strong; it offsets the blustery wind and the chill of the night.

Tom and Janis find that their time together in welcoming the seasons is peaceful and instructive. They have learned that nature is to be accepted and enjoyed; and, whenever they can directly experience its elegance and beauty, they bond with the Earth and feel closer to each other.

69. Roughing It

Expect the unexpected.

- ❦ 2 to 3 days (minimum) away from the comforts of home
- ❦ Appropriate gear
- ❦ Adequate preparation (highly recommended)
- ❦ Affiliation with guide or group (when necessary)

$\mathcal{I}$f there is a wild card in the game of love and romance, it has to be the overnight camping trip. It can be the source of great inspiration or disaster. A rendezvous with nature, a night beneath a star-studded sky, hiking and backpacking, breathing clean air, and sitting by a campfire all contribute to a renewed zest for life and living. The experience can deepen your appreciation for Mother Earth and, at the same time, teach you the true meaning of flexibility.

Then there are the unexpected challenges: excessive rain and mud, annoying campers nearby, faulty or insufficient gear, poison oak or ivy, tick attacks, the mosquito militia, or having your entire food supply ravaged by an uninvited animal guest. The ironic thing is that some of the worst camping trips produce the best memories. John, a camping enthusiast, put it this way, "If you are camping alone and everything is going wrong, you may want to just pack it in and go home. But, when you're with someone you love, there's a tendency for each of you to encourage the other to hang in there. It's *getting through it together* that promotes teamwork, very positive for any relationship, and makes the memory of an unpleasant camping experience so sweet."

If you are no stranger to camping, you are already familiar with many of its challenges and benefits. If you have never done it, or haven't in a long time, you may want to get some guidance and supplies from a local outfitter store — or visit Internet sites like hikingandbackpacking.com — to plan a two- or three-night venture. Consider seeking the advice of a guide, reading travel guide books about your area, or joining a small group of experienced enthusiasts — particularly if you are going to be backpacking in remote areas. If finances are a concern, you may be able to borrow some equipment from a friend or neighbor to minimize the initial cost of entry.

Cautionary note: Don't venture too far or too long from home on your earliest camping trips; pitch tent at nearby campgrounds or at a state park. Neophytes almost always forget important things like matches, bug repellent, hats, extra dry socks, and warm clothing. You don't want to be off in the middle of nowhere when that happens. Aside from the inconvenience or discomfort, it might set off a nasty argument: "But I thought *you* were going to bring the toilet paper."

If you are interested in upscale romantic camping where there are more activities and additional work and risk, check into a dude ranch or sign up for a cattle round-up. You can tame your camping trip entirely — yet still enjoy country comfort — by going to a wilderness or National Park hotel. Friends of ours in South Africa discovered a unique setting for their honeymoon: their "room" was a platform high up in a tree on a big gaming reserve!

Possible outcomes from Roughing It are as countless as the stars. Just realize they are rarely devoid of surprises, and you will almost certainly value the time away together. There is also the additional advantage of seeing how you and your partner act, as individuals and as a couple, when you are outside of your element. That alone could be worth the price of admission!

Sample Serving

Although they had known each other since childhood, Rolf and Alexia were newlyweds before Alexia agreed to follow Rolf blindly into a world that was so familiar to him and foreign to her: communing with the great outdoors.

August is the most likely time to find warm, sunny weather along the unpredictable Oregon coast. The young couple drove for three days, staying in charming oceanside motels as Rolf scouted for the perfect spot. He finally decided on a remote area by a lighthouse atop a jagged crumbling cliff. Alexia had never spent any time in a tent, let alone being perched upon a precarious bluff overlooking the vast, unbounded ocean. But standing beside her man with enough gear on his back to weigh down a team of mules, she looked at him with adoration and anticipation and contemplated their pending love affair with nature.

Knowing that Alexia might be apprehensive about her first camping experience, Rolf had come well prepared. He dropped the heavily laden pack from his shoulders, and out came the down pillows and comforter, sleeping bags, cooled champagne, a new hibachi, and a bag of coals that would soon be cooking their New York steaks. And, of course, there were slippers, a camera that would capture Alexia's first naked expression in nature, and the sweaters and layers of clothing that would make her first night warm and comfortable.

A delighted and innocent Alexia, who assumed that everyone geared up this way, helped Rolf set up camp. The light ocean breeze caressed and cooled their skin as they prepared their first meal together; their music was the sound of waves crashing against the rocks below. That night, and for the next few days, all they had was each other and there wasn't a single thing missing or wanting. Years later, after the accumulation of houses and other worldly things, Rolf would likely give it all up for a flimsy little tent perched high on a crumbling cliff, alone with that little girl who had grown into a woman and who sat with him enjoying the essence of simple caring love.

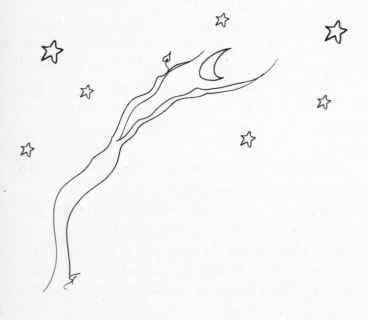

Beyond the Two of Us

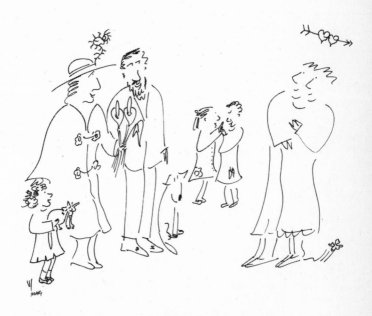

*Those who bring sunshine to the lives of
others cannot keep it from themselves.*

— James Matthew Barrie

70. Family Affair

Kids! If you can't avoid 'em, join 'em.

- ❧ Flexibility when you can't be alone
- ❧ Creativity in involving the whole family
- ❧ Ability to postpone desire

*L*eslie's mother once asked her dentist if he and his family had a wonderful vacation. "When my wife and I go alone, it's a vacation," he responded, "but with the kids, it's a trip."

Sound familiar, parents? Sometimes, when you're caught up in a Family Affair, it's difficult if not impossible to even think about being romantic. So what can you do when you really need to be alone but the kids need you more? Or they suddenly get sick? Or the babysitter cancels at the last minute or can't even be found?

We have four children and have had our share of setbacks, disappointments, and changes in plans. The trick, we've learned, is: one, accept it and understand it is going to keep on happening; and two, figure out ways for the kids to participate in the romance. Your children will love helping you make and hang decorations, and serving as go-betweens to deliver messages (as in the next recipe). Best of all, it will give them the opportunity to gain a healthy perspective on love and romance from their wonderful role models. In the early years of our relationship, we included our son, David, in a number of our romantic scenarios. Today he is a budding twenty-year-old romantic who gave us several excellent recipes for this book.

Romance delayed does not have to be romance denied. Keep the kids busy in activities that may tire them more quickly and help get them to bed earlier. Later, when they're asleep, you can make up for lost time. The anticipation may actually serve to heighten the enjoyment of your post-Family Affair tryst.

Sample Serving

Ann and Don could not find a babysitter to watch their three-year-old son, Ian, for Valentine's Day. So when Don and Ian went out together the day before, and then returned home empty-handed, Ann felt let down. She went to bed early with little to look forward to on what should have been her special day.

The next morning, Don left the house at dawn as he did every day. Ann was able to sleep in until 8:00 A.M., when she heard the patter of tiny feet in the hallway outside her room. Instead of jumping right into the bed, as Ann expected, Ian entered the room and boomed, "Open your eyes, Mommy.

Happy Valentine's Day. I love you so much and Daddy loves you even more!"

Ann opened her eyes, as instructed, but couldn't believe what she saw. There stood Ian holding a huge bouquet of red tulips that he and Don had hidden in a closet the night before. He smothered Ann with hugs and kisses before leading her into the kitchen, which had been transformed into a virtual Valentine. There were countless hearts, balloons, feathers, and streamers, in addition to love notes spelled out in Cheerios™. Ann saw only red and white everywhere she looked. At her spot at the breakfast table sat an exquisite red leather knapsack, which Ann has used almost every day since. In addition to its beauty and utility, it is a continual reminder of her "one in a million mornings."

71. The Go-between

A tried-and-true catalyst for love and intrigue!

- ❦ Trust in a third party
- ❦ Inclination to surprise
- ❦ 1 or more gifts (optional)

In romantic literature and drama, a trusted messenger is often used to relay oral or written messages between lovers and facilitate clandestine meetings. Often the communication is secret because the families or society would be opposed to such a reunion. In life, a go-between may be used for this purpose, or, ,ore commonly, to send out trial balloons of love from one person to anotyher because at least one of the parties is too shy, embarassed, or afraid to sit down and discuss his feelings. Either way, involving a third party can add a sense of flirtation or seduction to romance and make it more dramatic.

Even if you have a partner and don't need the services of a go-between, you may want to do it anyhow. Now and then, engage a friend, family member, or coworker to help set up or carry out a date that will catch your partner off guard. Examples are: relying on a confidante to get a romance started with someone you think is really hot; having your daughter deliver notes each day, written in advance, to your husband while you're out of town; and asking your wife's coworker to invite her to lunch and then drive her to meet you for some afternoon delight!

The better the go-between knows your partner, the better he can assist you in planning and pulling it off, as in recipe 25: The Pleasure List. Of course, an inept go-between like the bartender in recipe 18: Unforgettable may be a source of frustration at the time of the date, but his actions — or inaction — are part of the treasured memory.

Sample Serving

On one occasion while we were dating, I invited Jimmy to dinner at my house for a sensational meal and asked him to dress nicely for me. When he arrived, my son David met him at the door and told him he could not yet go into the kitchen. David took Jimmy into his room and entertained him as I slipped out through the back door and drove off.

Jimmy grew more curious about what was going on behind the kitchen door. After five minutes David doused him with cologne and gave him a card from me. The card invited Jimmy to find me "exactly where we were eight months earlier." David laughed as Jimmy searched desperately — first in the kitchen, then the bedroom, then throughout the house. Finally he counted back to Valentine's

Day, which had been one of our first dates together, and recalled our Italian feast at a beachside hotel.

I felt nervous and excited as I waited for Jimmy in the hotel lobby. I greeted him wearing the same dress I had on eight months earlier. Tears came to both of our eyes as Jimmy rushed inside to join me.

I loved treating us to dinner, and keeping the plans secret for the week before. Jimmy couldn't get over how well David (only nine at the time) did his part to help create such a beautiful, romantic evening.

72. Mum's the Word

*To be successful, your partner must
be the last one to know.*

- 🍎 1 special day expanded to fill several days
- 🍎 3 to 5 secret activities
- 🍎 Reliable confidantes

*P*lan a variety of secret activities with close friends, family, and coworkers to celebrate your loved one's birthday or another special occasion for several days. Your participants will probably have some of their own ideas for entertainment and will also enjoy plotting and scheming and keeping mum. Welcome their assistance. It will prevent you from burning yourself out in the process. Of course, be sure to keep any blabbermouths or tipsters out of the loop! And be mindful of your own gestures; even a change in the tone of your voice or a certain smile may tip her off.

If her birthday falls in the middle of the week, you may want to add an element of surprise by starting the weekend before, and staging different activities leading up to the actual day. You and your co-conspirators will find that the planning and the anticipation can be as rewarding as the events themselves.

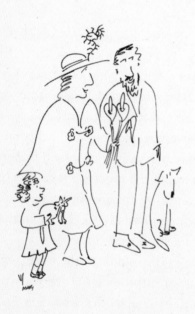

73. Talk of the Town

*The only thing sweeter than knowing we are loved
by many is hearing we are loved by many.*

- 1 secret time and location
- 1 guest list
- 1 anecdote per guest
- Refreshments or dinner
- Scribe and/or camcorder (highly recommended)

No one ever tires of sincere compliments, and one of the most dramatic and touching ways to honor your loved one is to arrange a surprise party where he will get lots of them from close family and friends. It can be done as part of a birthday or anniversary celebration, or stand on its own as a special evening of appreciation. Give each guest, who has had time beforehand to prepare what to say, a couple of minutes to reveal personal and complimentary anecdotes about your partner. Conclude the occasion with some amusing stories and a testimonial of your own.

Talk of the Town may be held at your own or someone else's home, a local club or restaurant, or may be staged as part of an outing or vacation. You can engage someone with good penmanship to write down all those wonderful compliments as a permanent keepsake; or, to capture the full emotion of the experience, be sure to bring a camcorder and videotape the occasion.

Sample Serving

Jimmy once found a novel way to honor me on my "birthday." One evening we picked up our son, David, from his karate lesson and walked to one of our favorite restaurants. As we went inside, I was amazed to see many familiar faces, balloons rising to the ceiling, and gifts piled on a table. Then I was showered with one "Happy Birthday" greeting after another from family members and friends.

Curious and confused, I turned to Jimmy. He informed me that this was the day I turned thirty-five and a half. It was a fun party that included crazy gifts like a cane, denture cream, a half-liter of wine, a half-dozen donuts, and a deck of playing cards with half the cards missing. I felt quite special by the way everyone made such a big deal out of my surprise celebration. Particularly touching were the things people said as they toasted me. Some were humorous, and others acknowledged my artistic talents, caring nature, and love of parenting.

I always marvel at Jimmy's ability to organize events and people without my knowledge. I'm lucky to have a man who's willing to go more than halfway!

74. Let's Party

Wow your friends with the right kind of spin;
they'll want to come back again and again.

- ❦ Desire to host or cohost
- ❦ Unique party theme
- ❦ Creative invitations and decorations
- ❦ Complementary games and activities

Many parties are held around the holidays, or on birthdays, anniversaries, and special occasions. You can add an innovative twist to your social scene by inviting people to your home for a romantic theme party. Examples are: a Valentine party where everybody wears red, sensuous wine-tasting by candlelight, adult or pajama party, aphrodisiac or dessert potluck, or a moonlit pool party.

You can lighten the responsibility by cohosting your theme party with another couple. Also, you might want to get creative with the invitations and decorations, and include games or activities that complement the theme. There are explanations of numerous games for all kinds of party themes at websites such as www.party411.com.

When a particular party is an overwhelming success, consider having it on an annual basis. We staged an elaborate Indian potluck dinner in our garden that was a rich sensory feast. It abounded in the smell of exotic spices, the sight of colorful costumes and umbrellas, and the sound of sitar music mixing with warm and friendly conversation. It was such a big hit that people kept asking when we could do it again. Now, every summer is initiated by that party in our household.

Of course, a terrific party provides the ideal atmosphere for relaxing and deepening friendships, and serves to create enjoyable times in the future when guests reciprocate your kindness. Life opens up when you open your house to entertain people in a way they will never forget.

75. The Secret of Living

What you keep is lost —
What you give is yours forever.

— S'hota Rustaveri

* Attitude of gratitude
* Compassion for those less fortunate
* Defined areas of giving

*G*iving. It's healthy. It's soulful. It's wonderful. Many individuals know the joy of sharing the wealth of their lives — time and money — with those less fortunate. For couples, it helps support romance because it keeps you in the spirit of giving; whenever you give to others, they benefit and you get back so much more. Even if you don't have a lot of money, there are a few simple things you can do to make a big difference in the lives of others.

Create a day for giving: Go to the bank and pick up a handful of one-dollar bills, or go to a fast-food restaurant and purchase gift certificates. Then, go to an area of town where you would expect to find people who could use some attention. Walk together down the street and offer your donations and a friendly ear to individuals who appear to be in need. You may be treated to a few fascinating stories. Just being a good listener may mean more to some people than anything else you could offer. Next, return home to clean out closets and the garage and bring your bags of unneeded stuff to your favorite charity thrift store. If you find some nice stuffed animals, take them to the pediatric ward of a nearby hospital. Afterward, be sure to relax or exercise before spending a quiet evening together. Reflecting on the day, you will feel prosperous, more appreciative of life, proud of your joint efforts and the way you have invested your time.

There are so many options for giving: Read to a blind person, serve dinner at a homeless shelter, bake Christmas cookies for the elderly who are homebound, deliver Valentine's Day treats to a friend who has recently ended a close relationship, help organize an Easter egg hunt for unfortunate children, stage or organize a yard sale to raise money for a worthy cause. Your local newspaper is a good source of charitable organizations that need volunteers on a one-time or continuing basis. We all lead busy lives, yet planning time for giving throughout the year will add to the goodness in the world and, as importantly, expand the heart. If you have children, be sure to find activities they can be included in. Let them learn early in life that they, too, can make a difference.

Getting involved with a charity whose objectives you

wholeheartedly support also creates the opportunity to meet other committed volunteers. Those who are giving, by nature, tend to make good friends. They think beyond themselves and want to help make this world a better place to live in.

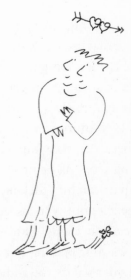

76. Friends for Life

True friendship is like good wine. It only gets better with time.

- ❦ Association with other loving couples
- ❦ Creation of opportunities for sharing and caring

One of the highest ideals of a strong, healthy love relationship is that each partner thinks of the other as "my best friend." Security and personal growth are strong and intact when you can count on your mate for unconditional support through thick and thin, for better and for worse. Outside friendships can never replace what you need from each other, but they can enrich your lives significantly. When you cross paths in life with people you are truly in sync with, it can be a lifelong source of joy.

Make it a priority to associate with other couples who are progressive and happy. They don't have to share your backgrounds or your politics, but they should reflect your interests and your values. In addition to socializing and having fun together, you get to compare notes and exchange ideas about male-female dynamics, parenting, gift giving, and romantic things to do. Some of the best humor and inspiration can come out of these recollections.

To make the best use of your time with other couples, don't limit your contact to evenings out for dinner and a show. Be sure to plan diverse vactivities that encourage as much interaction as possible. Some examples are: bowling parties, barbecues, reading and dinner clubs, theme parties with games, walking and hiking, tennis and golf. Vacationing and cruising are popular with many couples who are close, particularly when they live in different parts of the country. Meeting at a fascinating or exotic location is more relaxing for everyone because it spares one of the couples the pressure of being the hometown host and doing all the entertaining.

Remember, as you work and play together to strengthen your own relationship, be mindful of the company you keep. Your time is precious, so be sure to invest it with other loving couples. There's a lot of truth to the notion that your choice of people to hang out with says a lot about who you are.

Sample Serving

Robyn and Michael Bartling of Montecito, California, have made it a priority to develop close friendships with other couples who share their feelings about marriage and commitment. In each of the past ten years, they have staged wonderful celebrations on Valentine's Day as a way of honoring those friends and letting them know just how much they are appreciated. Robyn is responsible for the initial planning, and she exercises her creativity by trying to make each year's event distinct from all the previous ones.

She is especially proud of their celebration of Valentine's Day 2001: two couples received invitations to "a barefoot formal" at the Bartling's home. When the couples arrived, they were immediately blindfolded and chauffeured to a parking spot at the beach across from the Four Seasons Resort Santa Barbara. When the blindfolds were removed, the couples were flattered and excited to know they would be dining at the world-famous hotel.

Robyn and Michael smiled and told their guests they had planned to start the evening with a champagne toast on the beach. They all marveled at the beautiful candles lighting the stone stairway down to the beach; and once barefoot on the sand, they were equally intrigued by a string of tiki torches leading to a white tent that shimmered in the moonlight. They all agreed it must be the site of a Four Seasons wedding; and, at the suggestion of Robyn and Michael, they strolled over to take a closer look. The candle glow behind the closed curtains was too tempting. The couples peeked in to find a magical setting. There were candles and rose petals everywhere. In the middle was a round banquet table elegantly set with pink linens and china for six. It was time for Robyn and Michael to share their surprise. "Happy Valentine's Day. This is our gift to you."

Their spellbound guests were then served a five-course sit-down dinner. Earlier that day, Michael had prepared the meal and stored it in large coolers which had been hidden from view when they entered the tent. It included cold poached salmon with cucumber dill sauce, salad, and heart-shaped desserts and candies. Afterward, they opened the tent curtains, toasted each other, and drank champagne in the moonlight. As wave after wave crashed rhythmically against the shore, they delighted in acknowledging their friendship and making plans for the future.

Naughty 'n' Nice

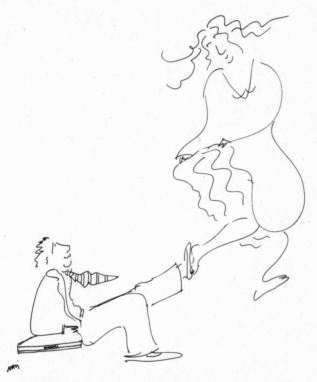

*When choosing between two evils I always like
to take the one I've never tried before.*

— Mae West

77. Pleasure Hunt

A homemade amorous adventure!

- ❦ Adequate time to plan
- ❦ 1 strong dose of imagination
- ❦ 3 to 5 clues
- ❦ 3 to 5 gifts
- ❦ 3 to 5 places to hide clues and gifts
- ❦ Helpful hands (optional)
- ❦ 1 mystery or romantic conclusion

*A*nytime, day or night. The setting can be your house, the neighborhood, or the city at large. Clues (and perhaps a few matching gifts) will delight and tease your partner as she is guided from one location to another. Friends may be involved to help along the way. Ideally, the hunt should lead to a big mystery present, or conclude with a secret rendezvous at a romantic hideaway. You can enhance the romantic effects of Pleasure Hunt by incorporating some imaginative exotic or erotic features.

Veronica found a novel way to celebrate gift giving with her boyfriend, Ted. On the morning of his birthday, she gave him a handmade birthday card that included a gift certificate from his favorite store. He was instructed to go there that morning and ask for a sales assistant named Megan. Ted met with Megan, who helped him buy a new shirt and encouraged him to wear it out of the store. Upon leaving, he was handed an envelope with another certificate directing him to see Kirk at a men's shop on the next block. Ted added trousers to his wardrobe with the assistance of Kirk, who sent him off to yet a third store with a certificate and instructions to see Rhonda. She helped complete his handsome outfit with the addition of socks and a leather belt.

Ted thoroughly enjoyed the flow of this gift giving game and all the personal attention he received. He was not surprised when Rhonda handed him his fourth and final envelope from Veronica. He smiled as he read, "Now that you're hot, birthday boy, get yourself to the Adult Store down the street and pick out something for me. Then come straight to my apartment to begin the real fun."

It was definitely a memorable birthday for the two of them.

78. Overexposed

Show and tell with a sizzle!

- ❦ 1 or more intimate apparel shops
- ❦ 1 dressing room large enough for two
- ❦ 2 doses of ambition without inhibition

*H*ere's something playful and totally outrageous to do with your hottie. If he's a reluctant shopper, assure him this is one outing he will not want to miss.

Visit one or more stores that offer intimate apparel for both men and women. Help each other make the sexiest selections of lingerie, bikini underwear, sexy silk robes or pajamas, then go into the dressing room together. Even if you don't end up buying anything, you'll love the time you spend modeling for each other.

If you're feeling a little self-conscious about doing this where you might be spotted, wait until you're out of town or on vacation. The hardest part of this recipe, of course, is controlling your behavior. Don't be surprised if you are overtaken by, among other things, excessive giddiness and laughter.

79. Light My Fire

Your partner's wish is thy command.

- 1 healthy serving of private time
- Freedom to express true desires (first partner)
- Unconditional surrender (second partner)
- Exotic costume (optional)

Give your partner the gift of freedom... to express her secret desires in a safe and supportive setting. Schedule at least several hours when the two of you can be alone without any interruptions or distractions. If you're going to be at home, be sure to prearrange outside babysitting for the children.

Encourage your lover to ask for what *really* turns her on. Your role is to be servant and confidant, responsive to each and every request, big or small: reading erotica, painting her toenails red, indulging in a food fantasy, sketching her in the nude, brushing her hair, reenacting a romantic scene from a favorite movie, making your own adult photos or videos. (With digital cameras and camcorders, you don't have to send anything out for developing.) Perhaps she longs for a lengthy foot rub or a full-body massage, or she wants to guide you in how to make love to her and participate in one of her sexual fantasies.

This level of intimacy is sure to promote open, honest communication and take your romance several notches higher. Don't be surprised if you learn new things about each other; you will probably share a lot of laughs, and, possibly, some tears. Also, if either one of you has been holding back in your communication in any way out of fear or inhibition, this recipe will leave you feeling lighter and more vibrant.

Sample Serving

Charles was really taken aback when he arrived home on the evening of his second anniversary. His wife, Charlotte, greeted him wearing a skimpy black-and-white maid's outfit and speaking with a delightful French accent. She told him that his wife had gone out for the evening, and that she had been hired to give him anything his heart desired.

He asked her to prepare a bath, and then massage his head, shoulders, toes, and thighs as he relaxed in the warm, soothing water. Afterward, she fed him, bite by bite, his favorite meal: eggplant parmigiana with garlic bread, Caesar salad, and a glass of Merlot. Throughout dinner, Charles was acting quite horny and couldn't keep his hands off Charlotte-turned-French maid. Afterward, though, he surprised her by asking her to accompany him, not to the bedroom, but to the office. He said he had forgotten some important papers that he needed for a meeting the next morning outside the office. Although it was getting late, she stayed in character and agreed.

The building in the heart of the city was quiet and seemed empty. Once inside the office, Charles led his French maid toward a familiar couch. They were kissing and touching each other so passionately, however, that they never made it that far. They dropped to the carpeted floor and started to undress each other. Thinking they had the building all to themselves, they didn't bother to restrain their voices or groans. Things were very hot and heavy when, suddenly, the door opened wide and the building's lone security guard shined his flashlight right at them, asking in a flustered voice if they were authorized to use the office after hours. Charlotte was totally embarrassed as she tried, ineptly, to cover herself. Charles, on the other hand, was nonchalant. "We're authorized," he responded, "but I don't know for how much longer."

This took place almost thirty years ago. Charles and Charlotte remain happily married, with wonderful children and grandchildren. Charles still chuckles when he reflects on the incident, adding that he got funny looks from almost everyone he passed in the office building for the next few months. It ended when he moved to a new office several blocks away where no one knew the story of what happened that night.

80. Body Heat

If it's getting too hot, you're in the right spot!

- 1 working fireplace
- Plenty of kindling and firewood
- All the time in the world
- Willingness to take things very slowly
- Generous supply of towels, blankets, and pillows
- Massage oil, light food and drink (recommended)

Just as there is an art to making a wonderful fire, there is an art to making love by the fire. In the event you have not given it too much thought before now, here are a few simple things you can do to maximize your pleasure in the perfect environment for physical intimacy.

First things first: You don't want to be rushed or disturbed. Allow for at least two hours, and make sure you will be the only ones at home during that time, with doors locked and phone ringer off. Next, decide on a few things you may want during your time together by the fire (massage oil, water, wine and cheese) and put them on the hearth or on a small table within easy reach. This eliminates the need to get up and possibly break the mood. The last stage of preparation is to make a cozy setting. Put down a soft covering such as a double-sized sleeping bag, one or two thick blankets, or a soft rug, and cover it with an oversized fluffy bath towel or a fresh sheet and soft pillows. Also, have a couple of extra towels or light blankets close at hand.

Meet by the hearth in bathrobes or loose-fitting attire and start the fire together. As it builds, sit back and watch the flames dancing; this is what our ancestors did before the advent of television. It can be very meditative. Do it in silence or engage in a good Heart-to-Heart (recipe 19). If you become hungry or thirsty, your solution is close at hand. As you sink into the warmth of the room and the affections of each other, one of you will want to get the massage oil and give your lover a foot, neck and shoulder, back, or full-body massage; then switch roles. Even though you are close to the fire, there still may be a draft in the room. This is when you'll appreciate having the extra towels and blankets.

You are now players in a multisensory show you have helped to create: the soothing heat, play of light, and crackling sounds coming from the fireplace; the aroma of massage oil mixed with the fragrant smell of wood burning; the gentle touch of loving hands releasing the tensions in your body; and the radiant beauty of your partner's skin in the glow of the fire. By this time, it will be hard to keep your passion in check; it will intensify like a fire burning out of control and lead you to the supreme pleasure of two souls coming together in perfect union. Afterward, you can prolong those wonderful feelings of intimacy by continuing to relax and cuddle together by the fire. If you're feeling drowsy, don't deny the sleep that follows. Stay there; or, at some point, get up and go to bed.

This fire-induced form of lovemaking is highly recommended for couples who want to achieve a high state of arousal through sensual sex. If you don't have a fireplace, spread a number of candles of varying heights across the floor; this, too, has its own unique charm. Or spend a night at a local hotel or bed-and-breakfast that has a fireplace in the room. If you're really adventurous, camp out next to a bonfire in a private outdoor area. You'll figure it out; and once you do, you'll be hooked!

81. Love Nest

The rainbow's end of romance.

- ❦ 1 uncluttered room (other than your bedroom)
- ❦ Freedom from dot.com and tele-everything
- ❦ Assorted flowers and candles
- ❦ 1 medley of scents or aromatherapy
- ❦ Romantic music

Optional

- ❦ 1 to 2 soft-colored lightbulbs
- ❦ 1 special set of sheets
- ❦ Erotic accessories
- ❦ 1 alternate site

*H*aving an alternate location for lovemaking away from the bedroom can free you from familiar trappings, and often invokes a sense of mystery or intrigue. Choose a room or location other than the bedroom that is free of clutter and electronic interference (computer, television, and telephone).

Your Love Nest should appeal to all the senses. Place fresh flowers around the room. Scented candles, incense, or a few drops of perfumed oils on pillowcases and soft-colored lightbulbs, can be used to heighten the atmosphere.

If you're feeling extravagant, buy a special set of red satin sheets just for the occasion and mist them with a scent that blends with other fragrances in the room (recipe 6: Two Scents' Worth).

Just before escorting your partner into your erotic sanctuary, put on your favorite romantic music to solidify the mood. Once inside, let the spirit of playfulness take over. You may want to experiment with erotic massage oil, Kama Sutra products, and natural aphrodisiacs like chocolate.

Some couples transform a spare room into a love den and use it for that purpose alone. Others create an ad hoc Love Nest in a quiet area of their home. In one town, several close friends rent an apartment and keep it a secret from everyone else. They take turns sneaking off to their hideaway, day or night. Each couple has their own closet to keep intimate apparel, books, videos, and erotica.

Love Nest provides an ideal setting for greater sexual freedom and expression. It can grow in charm and appeal as you add your personal touches to it over time. By its very nature, it is destined to produce some of your most cherished memories as lovers. Treat yourselves to this ultimate lap of luxury. Where there is a will, you will definitely find your way!

Kenny and Julia Loggins, who first suggested this recipe to us, combine it with regular Heart-to-Hearts (recipe 19) to create a Sacred Space in their marriage. They share the wonderful story about their "Big Sur love shack" in recipe 52.

82. Dressed for Sex-cess

Home alone, in style.

- ❧ 1 sexy outfit or X-rated costume
- ❧ Time to let the night unwind
- ❧ 1 heart-shaped pizza (optional)

*P*ick an evening when the two of you plan to spend an evening alone. Get home before your lover arrives, and early enough to greet him in an eye-popping, provocative outfit when he walks through the door. If he's already home, send him out on an errand, real or invented, so you can get into character. Lace, silk, and animal prints work well, particularly if it's something he's never seen on you before or couldn't imagine you wearing.

For a quick meal, contact a local pizza parlor the day before and arrange for a prepaid, heart-shaped pizza to be delivered at a certain time. Add a bottle of wine and a favorite dessert to complement the playful main dish. This recipe is one of the great appetite teasers. You can combine it with one of the previous recipes (Pleasure Hunt, Body Heat, Love Nest), or have it alone as a full-course meal.

83. Double Delicious

When breakfast in bed satisfies two appetites!

- ❦ 1 lazy morning
- ❦ Variety of aphrodisiacs
- ❦ Joyful expression of love

The word *aphrodisiac* is derived from the name of Aphrodite, the Greek goddess of love and beauty. The term has been used to describe anything — food, drink, drug, scent, or visual cue — that can stimulate or arouse sexual desire. Food, in particular, is often associated with romance because of its natural tendency to heighten sensory activity. Eating a sumptuous meal that incorporates foods known to stimulate libido can put you in a passionate mood for the lovemaking that follows.

Don't feel that romantic dining is restricted to lunch or dinner. A pre-planned breakfast in bed that includes delicious aphrodisiacs can take you and your lover to new heights of playfulness and pleasure, as well as get your day off to a beautiful start. On a lazy morning while your mate is still asleep, sprinkle rose petals on the pillows and sheets, or spray them with your favorite romantic scent (recipe 6: Two Scents' Worth). Quietly slip into the kitchen and prepare banana bread, a fruit salad, and strong hot coffee or green tea. The fruit salad should include at least some of the following: apples, grapes, figs, strawberries, papaya, mango, and oranges. For an added treat, the fruit can be dipped in warm chocolate sauce.

All of the above items have been acknowledged as sexual stimulants. You'll have more fun and feel less restrained eating together in bed if you plan to change the sheets that day and don't have to worry about being messy; or you can place an oversized soft cotton towel or washable blanket beneath you. For a real kick, take turns blindfolding and finger feeding each other samples from your menu (recipe 47: Finger Food). Mix up the tastes and see what surfaces as your preferred aphrodisiacs. You can spend the rest of the day evaluating their effectiveness!

This recipe lends itself to a lot of creativity, particularly when you become more knowledgeable about the relationship between food and romance. Paying closer attention to your diet and eating habits can play a significant role in the frequency of sexual delights. An excellent guide in this area is *Temptations: Igniting the Pleasure and Power of Aphrodisiacs* by Michael and Ellen Albertson.

Nate, an internationally trained chef and restaurant owner, loved to cook for his girlfriend, Samantha, and she loved to be cooked for. One night over dinner, she was caught off guard when he asked, "What would you like to be eating when I lick and kiss your naked body?" Intrigued by such a proposal, Samantha tried to imagine the perfect taste in such luscious circumstances. After a few minutes, she told Nate, "Warm sautéed peaches in a caramel *crème anglaise* sauce."

She thought it was just some kind of "What if?" game until Nate showed up at her door the next morning, holding a big, fuzzy, juicy, organic peach in each hand. At first, Samantha didn't make the connection; then, as she opened the door, it all clicked. She broke into a huge smile as Nate gave her a quick "hello" kiss and moved quickly to her tiny kitchen, where his professional training came in handy. Samantha thought there was little for him to work with, but sure enough, he put together a peachy dessert that exceeded her wildest expectations. And just as delightful as the taste was the way she got to eat it: reaching over beside the bed and feeding herself sticky pieces of ripe peaches with her fingers, at the same time she was enjoying marvelous stimulation from Nate's loving attention, touches, and kisses.

Samantha feels that life is made up of a series of memorable stories. She says that *two peaches* is one of her best.

Somewhere in Time

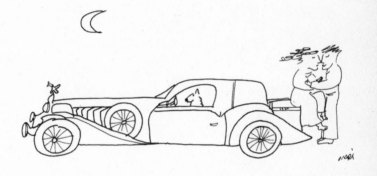

*Out of countless memories, invention selects a
few that become "the story of my life."*

— Mason Coole

84. Instant Replay

It's never too late to be young again.

- ☙ 1 special childhood memory
- ☙ Ability to bring the past forward on cue

There may be certain activities from your childhood that conjure up feelings of pure joy. Finding ways to reconnect with those experiences, bringing them into the present, and sharing them with the one you love is sweet for any relationship. Your partner will have access to the deeper chambers of your heart. She will know you more intimately and benefit from participating in your past.

The possibilities for Instant Replay are endless: it could be revisiting a school or campgrounds you loved as a child, or participating in a sport that was left behind in youth; it might be an activity you did every Saturday afternoon with a best friend, like seeing a double feature at the movies. There may have been a childhood hobby, like making motorized model airplanes and watching them fly. Perhaps there was a book or comic series your partner loved that the two of you could reread together.

Ed grew up and lives outside of Whistler, British Columbia, Canada. He was raised in a remote area by a lake. Every winter, he couldn't wait until the lake would freeze so he could watch his parents skating arm-in-arm. He still remembers the very first time he saw them; he was perched in a backpack on his grandfather's shoulders. His grandfather trekked around the lake on his snowshoes so young Ed could watch them perform. "They were ice dancers, all alone on the frozen lake."

The last time we spoke with Ed, he said a thin sheet of ice had formed over a nearby lake. In a day or two, he and Cathy, his wife of almost thirty years, would excitedly go skating arm-in-arm, something they had done many times over their years of marriage. The sweetness of Ed's youth remains alive for him and his wife to enjoy, and, as importantly, a beautiful family tradition continues.

85. Lovers' Lane

No matter where, it's the hottest street in town.

- 🍃 1 functioning car (the older the model, the better)
- 🍃 1 cassette or CD of rock 'n' roll music
- 🍃 Regression to high school behavior

Relive the fifties, sixties, seventies, or eighties. Make up any reason to take your partner somewhere. If possible, rent or borrow a car from that decade. Then drive to the beach or a quiet street and park. Pop in a cassette or CD of vintage rock 'n' roll and start necking. Be playful. Act as though you are back in high school. You'll soon discover how true it is: you're as young as you feel.

86. The Way We Were

God gave us memory so that we might have roses in December.
— James Matthew Barrie

- 2 open hearts
- Knack for nostalgia

*N*ow and then, get back in touch with those precious moments in your relationship by revisiting places from your past and reliving events. You may want to make periodic toasts to the time and way you met, commemorate significant days or turning points, or plan a unique reenactment of a treasured moment that may turn out to be as memorable as the original event.

Sample Serving

Mike and Angie were excited about celebrating their first anniversary at the bed-and-breakfast where they spent their honeymoon. It was a Southern mansion on many acres, reminiscent of *Gone with the Wind,* Angie's all-time favorite book and movie. Angie had several conversations with the owners of the B&B to make sure all her expectations could be met.

The big day finally arrived. Angie had packed their suit-cases and prepared snacks for the gorgeous drive through the antebellum South. Entering the front door of the mansion revived strong feelings of love and happiness for both of them. Everything was as beautiful as they remembered: the marble foyer and grand staircase, the smell of gardenias, sun-filled rooms with gleaming antiques, and, of course, the unequaled southern hospitality. They enjoyed the honey-moon suite the entire afternoon. When the cocktail hour began, Angie asked Mike to go downstairs while she finished getting ready for dinner. By 6:45 P.M., Mike was sitting at the same table they shared on their wedding night and nurs-ing a mint julep as he awaited his wife of exactly one year. At 7:00 P.M., the pianist began to play Wagner's "Wedding March" (Here Comes the Bride). Tears came to everyone's eyes as they saw Angie gliding down the staircase in her wed-ding dress and veil. Mike and Angie held hands throughout their candlelit dinner and relished the acknowledgments from other diners. Another couple was so happy for them that they sent over a bottle of champagne with a note that read, "Congratulations. Next year, two bottles!"

After dinner, Mike and his bride went outside to take in the warm evening air. They sat on a garden swing beneath the magnolia trees, reflected on their first year of marriage, and talked about their plans for the future. When they finally returned to the suite, Mike had a surprise of his own for Angie: a first edition of *Gone with the Wind*.

87. Name That Tune

A piece of the American pie.

- 1 or more favorite tunes
- 2 pairs dancing shoes
- 1 prearranged agreement with local band or deejay
- 1 long car ride (optional)
- Call to radio station request line (optional)

*T*ake your partner dancing at a night club where you have arranged beforehand for the band or disc jockey to play her favorite song or your favorite song as a couple. Or, before taking a long ride in the car, call a local radio station that takes requests and ask the deejay to dedicate that song to the one you love.

Sample Serving

When we went out one evening, I couldn't understand why Jimmy brought me to a smoke-filled bar. It definitely wasn't our kind of place. We walked to the dance floor in the back, where he introduced me to his friend Bruce, a one-man band on the keyboards. After some small talk, Jimmy coaxed me onto the dance floor. My knees weakened and I started to tremble as Bruce began the set with "Goin' Outta My Head." That song had been my number one hit as a teenager.

As Jimmy swept me across the dance floor, I realized it was the first time I had ever danced to this song. What a perfect combination: dancing to my old-time favorite with my all-time favorite.

88. The Possible Dream

The things we regret in life are never the things we did,
but the things we don't do.

— Herb Cohen, *Winning the Negotiating Game*

- ❧ 1 cherished dream
- ❧ Courage to overcome procrastination
- ❧ 1 involved partner

It's a feeling we all know. Someone or something makes such a deep impression on us that a desire, much like a little seed, begins to germinate in our soul. That desire can become so compelling that life just doesn't seem as if it will ever be complete without its fulfillment. It might mean meeting your favorite entertainer, reconnecting with an old friend after many years, buying a vintage car, vacationing on an exotic island, or living in a foreign country.

One of the great benefits of cashing in on a dream is that it eliminates a nagging thought that may keep coming up, "I always wanted to do that but never got around to it." And it can be even more satisfying, and quite romantic, when the experience is shared with a loved one. In fact, it may take the chemistry of a particular relationship to give you that final push toward fulfillment.

Sample Serving

Lori Ann was twenty years old when she sailed into Avalon Harbor at Catalina Island, California, and had her first glimpse of the famous Casino Ballroom. She felt an immediate connection with its magnificent rotunda perched majestically just above the ocean. While reading everything available on this architectural masterpiece, with its 180-foot circular ballroom, she learned about the definitive romantic event held there annually: a grand ball on New Year's Eve. She fantasized for years about the day when she and her perfect partner would be among the six hundred guests.

Twenty-six years later she met Steve and knew he would be the man to share her dream. As a way of celebrating their first year together, they planned a trip to Catalina for New Year's Eve, 2001, and were able to obtain coveted tickets to the grand ball. When the big day arrived, the weather forecast was discouraging for all flights going in and out of Santa Barbara, where they lived, and it appeared their plans might be in jeopardy. Lori Ann made several frantic calls to the ferry in Long Beach and realized there might be enough time to drive there and catch the last boat to Catalina. They arrived just in time; and several hours later, she and Steve checked into the five-star, "old-world charm" Metropolitan Hotel, where they could finally relax and get ready for the night of a lifetime.

The moon was full and shimmering on the water, as if guiding Lori Ann and Steve on their stroll along the old boardwalk from the hotel to the ballroom. As they made their entrance, Lori Ann thought she was stepping out of her fairy-tale dream and into a fairy-tale reality. She felt like a princess in her Max Mara silk gown, arm-in-arm with her handsome prince in his tuxedo. Elegantly dressed couples of all ages seemed to glide across the polished wooden dance floor beneath the sparkling glow of art deco chandeliers and soft candles. As she and Steve began to dance to the rich sounds of the sixty-piece orchestra, Lori Ann was happy she had waited for the right time with the right man to make her dream come alive.

89. Conversation Piece

What you get is more than what you see!

- 1 or more objects with a romantic history
- Obvious locations
- Knack for storytelling

Every relationship has its unique history, with special memories that couples like to reflect on and sometimes share with close friends and family. You can commemorate at least a part of your past by displaying art, unusual objects, furnishings, or memorabilia that are directly associated with your most romantic experiences. Place them in areas where they will be noticed by visitors to your home. The more unusual or striking an item is, the more you will be asked about the history behind it. Cautionary note: If you are not asked, do not direct your guests' attention to an item and volunteer information about it. A good host does not boast!

Sample Serving

One of the most romantic periods of our marriage was the two years we lived with our family in Italy. At the beginning of our last month there, we realized we had to bring some-thing home that captured the magic of our European stay. We decided on the item and made a special trip on Mother's Day to the Venetian island of Murano to custom design a handblown glass chandelier. When visitors drop by for the first or second time and spot this magnificent piece of art-work, we are often asked about the history behind it. This always brings a smile to our faces; we never tire of reminisc-ing about those wonderful times in Italy.

90. Love, American Style

Where junk food is the preferred menu.

- ❦ 1 drive-in movie theater
- ❦ 1 carload of food, pillows, and blankets
- ❦ 2 pairs of pajamas (highly recommended)
- ❦ Scenic area (alternative setting)

*S*urprisingly, many happy couples we interviewed for this book had never been to a drive-in movie together, or hadn't been to one since they started dating years ago. It's time to go again! Although the drive-in has become an endangered species, you can find a complete listing of locations, openings, and events on the web at drive-ins.com. Type in your zip code and it will give you a listing of all the drive-ins that are closest to you.

Remember to bring your favorite junk food, pillows or cushions, and blankets — no kids or friends. For a real kick, come in your pajamas and sit on the hood of your car or in the back of a pickup; recline on the pillows or cushions and cuddle beneath the blankets as you watch the movie. When you notice the steamy windows of the cars around you, it may inspire you to fool around like you were teenagers again!

If you live in an area that is too far from the closest drive-in, do a drive-out. Take a ride on a country or mountain road at sunset — with the food, pillows, and blankets, of course! — and stop at a scenic area. Watch and listen to the night. Let the moon and stars or the lights of the city be the feature presentation.

91. Déjà Food

A revival of the milk and cookies of youth.

❧ Access to your partner's food bank of memories
❧ Ability to deliver the past on a platter

Some of our deepest impressions from childhood revolve around food. You may not know everything that makes your partner tick, but one sure way to turn her on is to recreate a savory snack, dish, or meal she cherished as a child. It might be something you become aware of when she reflects on her early years, or a recipe you learn about from a close friend or relative. See if you can find a way to approximate the experience if you can't duplicate it.

There is an old saying: we are what we eat. Whenever you facilitate a reunion between your loved one and a tasty part of his past, you are bringing him back home. A treasured recipe may even be a direct link to a deceased relative or represent a strong connection to his heritage. Surprising your partner with a serving of Déjà Food will most certainly stir up feelings of emotional warmth and comfort.

Jimmy's Aunt Martha holds a special place in the hearts of everyone who knew her. An incessant talker, she had a huge heart and showed tremendous interest in everything she did and everyone she met. Visiting her was always a special treat. Whenever Jimmy and his family dropped by, Martha would always take out some of her delicious sour cream chocolate chip coffee cake and serve it along with her unconditional love.

When Kian, our fourth child, was born, Jimmy's sister surprised us by baking Aunt Martha's famous coffee cake for a welcome-to-the-world party. Unknown to us, she had queried Martha about the recipe over several conversations and recorded it just right for posterity. Everyone at the party raved about the cake so much that Leslie got the recipe and made it for Jimmy on a later occasion. He was so touched by the fond memories of being around Martha and her family that he asked Leslie if she would make the cake whenever they entertained close friends. Since that time, many people have visited our home and heard wonderful stories about Aunt Martha. They can almost feel her love as they taste each bite. Many guests — including a professional food critic — have left the house adoring a woman they never met and asking that the recipe be e-mailed or faxed to them.

In the spirit of Martha's giving nature, we offer her recipe and hope it will add a special touch of sweetness to your life as well.

Aunt Martha's Coffee Cake

1 cup sugar
$^1/_2$ pint sour cream (1 cup)
$^1/_4$ lb. butter
2 eggs
1 tsp. vanilla
2 cups flour
1 tsp. baking soda
1 tsp. baking powder

Filling (to be mixed together):

$^1/_2$ cup brown sugar, packed
1 cup chocolate chips
   (can be increased to 2 cups for chocolate lovers)
$^1/_2$ cup chopped nuts
   (can be increased to 1 cup for nut lovers)

Sift flour, then measure and sift again with baking soda and baking powder.

Cream the butter and sugar, add eggs and sour cream. Add dry ingredients and vanilla.

Cooking Tip: Have the eggs at room temperature and add them one at a time. (Mix the first one into the batter, then add the second one.)

Grease 9-inch tube pan and add $1/2$ the batter, sprinkle with $1/2$ the filling; add the rest of the batter. Put the rest of the filling over the top.

Bake in 350° oven for 45–50 minutes. Start testing at 40 minutes.

When the cake is ready, let it cool for a few minutes and then turn it onto a cooling rack. Immediately turn it over again onto another cooling rack so that the nut and chocolate chip mixture is on top of the cake.

This cake freezes well. Aunt Martha always had some in the freezer for any guests who might drop by.

P.S. We hope the recipes in this book will serve to enrich your romantic life and bring you much satisfaction. They have worked for so many couples already that we are certain they can work for you. Always remember: Whether you are rich or poor, famous or obscure, outgoing or shy, sought-after or forgotten, you are as capable of loving and being loved as any other person in this world. What goes around comes around, and love is no exception! So open your heart. Speak your love today!

Acknowledgments

This book might never have surfaced were it not for the suggestions and heartwarming stories of the many people who are revealed in its pages. We are indebted to you for your time and interest in helping to make *Ready for Romance* as good as it could possibly be. We are doubly grateful to friends and family members who served as ad hoc advisors, editors, and cheerleaders along the way, particularly Rick Eisenberg, Hermine Hilton, Stewart Nurick, Justin Grant, Nicole Lacks, and David Caplan. Of course, having editors who push and challenge and cajole is a real plus for any creative project, and we thank Georgia Hughes and Kevin Bentley at New World Library for giving us the freedom to do anything, as long as it wasn't mediocre. Speak your love today!

About the Authors

Leslie & Jimmy Caplan were married in 1992 during one of their romantic getaways in Istanbul, Turkey. In addition to writing together and home schooling their three youngest children, the Caplans are engaged in various home-based endeavors. Leslie is an artist, currently concentrating on mosaics. Jimmy is an entrepreneur and motivational speaker, specializing in the areas of communication and negotiation. Together, they have developed their interest in coffee into a web-based business, www.romanticblends.com. The Caplans reside in Santa Barbara, California. They welcome your comments and suggestions for additional recipes for romance and can be contacted at www.readyromance@aol.com.